U0295781

国学经典外译丛书（第一辑）

伤寒论英译

On Cold Damage

〔东汉〕张仲景 ◎ 著

刘希茹 ◎ 今译　　李照国 ◎ 英译

上海三联书店

"十三五"国家重点图书出版规划项目

国家出版基金资助项目

达于上下 敬哉有土

——译事感怀

国学者，天人相应之积成，天人交融之精诚，天人合一之大成。盘古开天，国学与天地并生；伏羲造易，国学与六合并韵；炎黄树人，国学与三才并举；三代立本，国学与百族并融；秦汉统制，国学与万邦并荣。今日之高丽、扶桑、交趾，即其明证是也。

此非鄙人之见也，实乃历朝学人之志也、历代国人之意也。其志者，非梦也，非幻也，实乃春华秋实之景也；其意者，非妄也，非狂也，实乃天晴日明之象也。自三代以至汉唐，国学之神韵、国文之形意、国体之本末，皆悉传入中土之邻邦。其传者，非国人之意也，实异族之愿也。岁岁年年，高丽、扶桑、交趾，遣汉使，遣唐使，遣宋使，遣明使，跋山涉水，奔波神州。其行者，非劫财也，非谋利也，皆潜心研国学，习国文，求国典，由此而开辟夷人传承国学之坦途、光大国文之路径、珍储国典之金匮。

今日高丽所谓之韩医，扶桑所谓之汉方，交趾所谓之越医，皆随国学国文而传入之国医国药也。值此所谓之现代世界，国医于夷地，其形神意趣，则依然如故。其纯真，其淳朴，一如千秋万代之国学、国文与国医。自夏至清，中土虽时有改朝之举，虽偶有亡国之恨，然国学、国文与国医，则始终未因之而易，更未因之而亡。此态此势，非国人以命守之，实夷人以心继之。夷人既亡大汉之国，既立本族之邦，何以"继"大汉"往圣之绝学"？"木铎起而千里应，席珍流而万世响"，即其绝世之因由也。国学既"写天地之辉光"，既"晓生民之耳目"，自然感夷人而化夷邦，融百族而合万国。

惜哉！大明亡而大汉崩，大清衰而大汉丧！自鸦片之战，泰西列强，一如六淫七邪，借大清衰亡之际，侵入中土，劫江河，毁山川，破原野,欲攻赤县而灭神州。华夏之三才,由此而崩裂,炎黄之子孙,因此而昏聩。自此以来,反孔者,疑道者,日千千而年万万。时至今日,崇洋者,媚外者,已非千千万万,实乃举国上下。何以见之?"洋装"谓之"正装",可谓不言自明矣。"洋装"谓之"正装","国装"何以谓之?"斜装"也?"邪装"也?何人可以告知?何人可以明之?

国医于高丽、扶桑,至今依然淳朴,依然纯真,此与其"国装"为"正装"之心境,自然一一而相应,时时而对应。国人以"洋装"为"正装",其国医自然难以淳朴,难以纯真。其国学,自然难以传承,难以光大,甚或亦趋绝矣。国学之绝,何以见之?所谓"正装"者,皆系形之以形者也。而以夷人之教代之以儒道,则系神之以神者也。夷人之形,自有"直方大"之趣矣。其直形,其方形,其大形,可鉴可取,自然而然。荀子所谓之"善假于物",即言此矣。夷人之教也,乃其祖之传,其宗之缘,国人理应知之,理应明之,此乃彼此相尊相敬是也。恰如邻人之父母,彼此知之敬之,共和同合。所谓"远亲不如近邻",即言此举之要也。彼此虽相尊相敬,然彼之父母皆彼之父母,绝非此之父母,岂能取而代之!此理可谓人人知之,然其理之上者,其理之下者,却并非人人知之,更非人人明之。

如今中土之国医,皆遍布泰西之盗汗;神州之国药,皆洞穿西洋之涎沫。其历来之精气神韵,皆若寒冬腊月之日辉,明而无温,亮而无暖。此皆系传夷人之教、行夷人之理、遵夷人之道之故尔。国学乃国医之根,国文乃国药之本。国学绝矣,国医何以行健?国文异矣,国药何以载物?今日之神州,仰观而无吐曜,俯察而无含章。其故不辨自明矣。倘若"君子终日乾乾",国人何以至此?"黄河之水天上来",其水虽黄矣,必自然矣。所谓"天聪明,自我民聪明",即言此矣。倘若"黄河之水泰西来",其水虽清矣,然必毒矣。之所以毒矣,皆因化学元素变幻之故尔。今日闹市所售之诸水,即化学变幻之象尔,其毒矣,可谓无人不知,无人不晓。

自明晰天理以来,鄙人常告知友人学子,人人皆有两系基因,一则生理,与生俱来,无需求索。二则文化,全凭自力,仅求索而不可得,唯

达于上下　敬哉有土

修身而方可具。惜哉！此理虽可人人知之，然身处物化时代，何人甘愿自修、自取、自得？

以译事观之，则学界国之意识、民之见识、我之胆识，可谓淡而无象矣。国人之"龙"，谓之始祖。"龙之传人"，即谓此矣。然不知何人、何时、何因、何意，竟以泰西之 dragon 对译国人之"龙"。泰西所谓之 dragon，非华夏始祖之"龙"矣，实乃恶邪也，豺狼也。西人所谓之 monster，即喻 dragon 是矣。故而以 dragon 译"龙"，即以恶邪之喻神州也；以 descendants of dragon 译"龙之传人"，即以鬼魅之喻国人也。若神州为邪恶，若国人为鬼魅，岂能善乎夷人？岂能和乎异族？鄙人曾呼学界、译界、政界，明其善恶，辨其是非，除其正反。惜哉！时至今日，山依然高，水依然深。

自鸦片之战至今，泰西之言、文、学、教，一如今日之雾、霾、沙、尘，铺天盖地攻九州，山呼海啸陷神州。如今之举国上下，皆谓泰西之 Bible"圣经"，皆谓西洋之 Christmas"圣诞"，即其明证是也。某冬日时节，我为台胞授课，恰逢西洋之 Christmas，课间学子拱手谓之曰："耶诞快乐！"吾闻之不禁慨然，随问之曰："何以谓 Christmas 耶诞矣？"学子曰："吾等皆国人也。国人之'圣诞'，唯孔子之诞辰是也。"吾闻之，面红而耳赤，心酸而气滞。课后离席，魂消魄散，愧羞难已。自此以来，我以此为症痕，时常告诫学人学子。然所获者，唯子乎者也是矣。

惜哉！惜哉！

《淮南子》曰："以中制外，百事不废；中能得之，则外能收之。"此"中"若喻之"中土"，此"外"若喻之"外夷"，则国人将因之而"知所先后，则近道矣"。此乃鄙人译解《内经》《难经》之所感也，译释《伤寒》《金匮》之所悟也。此感此悟，非偏异之见也，实举目之望也，侧耳之闻也，扪心之问也，刻骨之切也。

李照国
丙申年五月初十于华亭

凡 例

1. 本译本以上海科学技术出版社出版的《伤寒论译释》为基础,并参考了历朝历代以及现代诸家的释本。

2. 译文每节文字包括三个部分,即"原文"、"今译"和"英译","今译"是用白话文对"原文"的释义,在此基础上将其译为英文。

3. 译文原则上以原文的文字结构和表达形式为基础,因表达需要而增加的英文单词或句子均附在方括号[ ]之中。

4. 译文中有些概念或术语出于对原文结构的传承,以直译或音译的形式予以表达,但对其实际含义则以圆括号( )的形式附录于后,作为文内注解。

5. 原文基本概念和术语原则上在译文中保持统一。但有时虽然是同一个概念和词语,但其含义则因背景的不同而有所变化,所以译文也有所调整。

6. 根据中医基本名词术语国际标准化的发展趋势,本书的所有剂量单位均采用音译,个别采用意译,基本形式和释义如下:

传统剂量单位	公制剂量单位	音译(或意译)形式
石	60 公斤	*dan*
斤	500 克	*jin*
两	31.25 克	*liang*
钱	3.125 克	*qian*
分	0.3125 克	*fen*
朱	1.3 克	*zhu*
斗	2 公升	*dou*

传统剂量单位	公制剂量单位	音译(或意译)形式
升	200 毫升	*sheng*
合	20 毫升	*ge*
钱匕	1.5—1.8 克	*qianbi*
方寸匕	5 毫升	*fangcunbi*
枚	颗、粒、片	*piece*

7. 中药和方剂名称的翻译,采用"四保险"的方式,以保证译文不出现任何差错,因为汉语同音字比较多。所谓"四保险",即音译之后以括号形式附以中文、英文和拉丁文。如"人参"译为：Renshen（人参, ginseng, Radix Ginseng）。

8. 中文的"龙",英文常译作 dragon,显然很不符合实际。"龙"是中华民族最具代表性的传统文化之一,而 dragon 则是西方人想象中的邪恶动物。所以西方对华友好的汉学家明确反对将"龙"译作 dragon,建议予以音译。所以本书将"龙骨"译作：Longgu（龙骨, Loong bone, Os Loong）,而不译作 Longgu（龙骨, dragon bone, Os Draconis）。

目 录

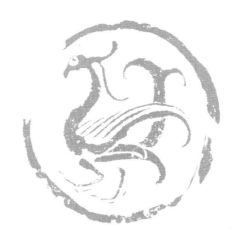

辨太阳病脉证并治上

【原文】

（一）

太阳之为病，脉浮，头项强痛而恶寒。

【今译】

太阳病，以脉象浮、头痛、项部强痛及畏寒为基本特征。

【原文】

（二）

太阳病，发热，汗出，恶风，脉缓者，名为中风。

【今译】

太阳病，有发热、出汗、恶风、脉象浮缓的症状，称为中风。

【原文】

（三）

太阳病，或已发热，或未发热，必恶寒，体痛，呕逆，脉阴阳俱紧者，名为伤寒。

【今译】

太阳病，已经发热，或者尚未发热，必然恶寒、身体疼痛、呕逆、阴阳脉象（即尺脉和寸脉）均浮紧，称为伤寒。

Differentiation of pulse and syndrome / pattern
[related to] taiyang disease and treatment (part 1)

Differentiation of pulse and syndrome/pattern [related to] taiyang disease and treatment (part 1)

【英译】

Line 1

Taiyang disease [is characterized by] floating pulse, stiffness and pain of the head and nape, and aversion to cold.

【英译】

Line 2

Taiyang disease, [characterized by] fever, sweating, aversion to wind and moderate pulse, is called wind stroke.

【英译】

Line 3

Taiyang disease, [characterized by] fever or no fever, aversion to cold, generalized pain, nausea, vomiting, and tight pulse of both yin and yang (chi pulse and cun pulse), is called cold damage.

【原文】

(四)

伤寒一日,太阳受之,脉若静者,为不传。颇欲吐,若躁烦,脉数急者,为传也。

【今译】

伤寒病发生的第一天,传入太阳。如果脉象静,说明没有传变。如果患者急于呕吐,身心烦躁,脉象数急,说明已经传变。

【原文】

(五)

伤寒二三日,阳明少阳证不见者,为不传也。

【今译】

伤寒病发作两三天后,若不见阳明、少阳病的症状,表示病未传变。

Differentiation of pulse and syndrome/pattern [related to] taiyang disease and treatment（part 1）

【英译】

Line 4

[In] the first day of cold damage，the taiyang [meridian] is attacked，the pulse is quiet and [the disease will] not be transmitted [to another meridian]. [If the patient is] nauseated and restless，and the pulse is rapid and tight，[the disease] will be transmitted [to another meridian].

【英译】

Line 5

[In] two or three days of cold damage，[if] yangming and shaoyang syndromes/patterns do not appear，[it] will not be transmitted [to another meridian].

【原文】

（六）

太阳病，发热而渴，不恶寒者，为温病。若发汗已，身灼热者，名风温。风温为病，脉阴阳俱浮，自汗出，身重，多眠睡，鼻息必鼾，语言难出。若被下者，小便不利，直视失溲。若被火者，微发黄色，剧则如惊痫，时瘛疭。若火熏之。一逆尚引日，再逆促命期。

【今译】

太阳病，有发热口渴、不恶寒的症状，就称为温病。如果使用发汗方法以后，身热如同烧灼一样，则称为风温。风温病的症候是阴阳脉（即尺脉和寸脉）都有浮象，不自觉出汗，身体沉重，经常睡眠，呼吸时鼻有鼾声，语言困难。假若误用下法，就会引起小便不利，两眼直视，小便失禁。假若误用火法，轻则导致皮肤发黄，重则引起类似惊痫的症状，手足时时抽搐痉挛。假若使用火熏之法，后果更加严重。首次误用治法，虽然使病情严重，却不会导致死亡。但若再次误治，就会危及生命。

Differentiation of pulse and syndrome / pattern [related to] taiyang disease and treatment (part 1)

【英译】

Line 6

Taiyang disease, [characterized by] fever, thirst and no aversion to cold, is called warm disease. If [there are symptoms and signs of] sweating and scorching heat, it is called wind-warm [disease]. The disease caused by wind-warmth [is characterized by] floating pulse of both yin and yang (chi pulse and cun pulse), spontaneous sweating, heaviness of the body, somnolence, snoring sound [in sleep] and difficulty in speech. If [the formula for] purgation is used, dysuria, staring vision and urine incontinence [will be caused]. If [the formula for] scorching is used, slight yellowing, convulsion and epilepsy [in acute cases] and periodic spasm will occur, as if being fumigated by fire. [There are] still a few days left for healing after the first time of adverse [treatment]. [But there will be] no time left for healing [if] adverse [treatment is used] again.

【原文】

（七）

病有发热恶寒者，发于阳也；无热恶寒者，发于阴也。发于阳，七日愈，发于阴，六日愈，以阳数七、阴数六故也。

【今译】

患外感病的，如果有发热畏寒症状的，属病在阳经；如果有无热畏寒症状的，属病在阴经。病在阳经的，一般七天可以痊愈；病在阴经的，一般六天可以痊愈。原因在于七属于阳数、六属于阴数。

【原文】

（八）

太阳病，头痛至七日以上自愈者，以行其经尽故也。若欲作再经者，针足阳明，使经不传则愈。

【今译】

太阳病，患者头痛至七日以上而自愈的，是因为完全传入其经。如果再传入他经，通过针刺足阳明经，可阻止其传入，从而使患者得以痊愈。

【原文】

（九）

太阳病，欲解时，从巳至未上。

【今译】

太阳病将要解除的时间，一般从巳时（上午 9 时至 11 时）到未时（下午 1 时至 3 时）。

Differentiation of pulse and syndrome / pattern
[related to] taiyang disease and treatment (part 1)

【英译】

Line 7

The disease with [the symptoms of] fever and aversion to cold originates from yang [aspect]; while the disease without [the symptoms of] fever and aversion to cold orginates from yin [aspect]. [The disease] originating from yang [aspect will be] healed in seven days, [while the disease] originating from yin [aspect will be] healed in six days, because the number of seven [pertains to] yang [while] the number of six [pertains to] yin.

【英译】

Line 8

Taiyang disease with headache that heals automatically over seven days is due to [the fact that it] transmits all through the meridian. If [the disease] tends to transmit to another meridian, [application of] acupunctures [treatment to the stomach meridian of] foot-yangming [will prevent it and] heal [it].

【英译】

Line 9

To subside taiyang disease, [it usually starts] from si (9:00—11:00) to wei (13:00—15:00).

【原文】

(一〇)

风家,表解而不了了者,十二日愈。

【今译】

太阳中风的患者,表证解除后,身体仍感不适者,十二日后则可痊愈。

【原文】

(一一)

病人身大热,反欲得衣者,热在皮肤,寒在骨髓也;身大寒,反不欲近衣者,寒在皮肤,热在骨髓也。

【今译】

患者全身有大热,但却想多穿衣服,因为热在皮肤,寒在骨髓。身体有大寒的患者,反而不想多穿衣服,原因是寒在皮肤,热在骨髓。

【原文】

(一二)

太阳中风,阳浮而阴弱。阳浮者,热自发,阴弱者,汗自出。啬啬恶

Differentiation of pulse and syndrome / pattern [related to] taiyang disease and treatment（part 1）

【英译】

Line 10

The disease caused by wind will heal in twelve days [when] the external symtoms is resolved but [the patient still feels] uncomfortable.

【英译】

Line 11

The patient with high fever but still in need of [putting on] more clothes [indicates that] heat is in the skin [while] cold is in the marrow. [If there is] cold in the body but [the patient] does not want to put on more clothes，[it indicates that] cold is in the skin [while] heat is in the marrow.

【英译】

Line 12

Taiyang [disease with] wind stroke [is characterized by] floating of yang（*chi* pulse）and weakness of yin（*cun* pulse）. Floating of yang [indicates] spontaneous fever [while] weakness of yin [indicates] spontaneous sweating. [The patient with] severe cold，aversion to cold and fever [as well as] snoring and nausea can be treated by Guizhi Decoction（桂枝汤，cinnamon twig decoction）.

Guizhi Decoction （桂 枝 汤，cinnamon twig decoction） [is composed of] 3 *liang* of Guizhi（桂枝，cinnamon twig，*Ramulus Cinnamomi*）（remove the bark），3 *liang* of Shaoyao（芍药，peony，Radix Paeoniae），2 *liang* of Gancao（甘草，licorice，Radix Glycyrrhizae Praeparata）（broiled），3 *liang* of Shengjiang（生姜，

寒,淅淅恶风,翕翕发热,鼻鸣干呕者,桂枝汤主之。

桂枝汤方

桂枝三两(去皮,味辛热)、芍药三两(味苦酸,微寒)、甘草二两(炙,味甘平)、生姜三两(切,味辛温)、大枣十二枚(掰,味甘温)。

右五味,[哎]咀。以水七升,微火煮取三升,去滓,适寒温,服一升。服已须臾,啜热稀粥一升余,以助药力,温覆令一时许,遍身,微似有汗者益佳,不可令如水流漓,病必不除。若一服汗出病差,停后服,不必尽剂;若不汗,更服,依前法;又不汗,后服小促其间,半日许,令三服尽;若病重者,一日一夜服,周时观之。服一剂尽,病证犹在者,更作服;若汗不出者,乃服至二三剂。禁生冷、粘滑、肉面、五辛、酒酪、臭恶等物。

【今译】

太阳中风症,阳脉浮而阴脉弱。阳脉浮的,自有发热。阴脉弱的,自会汗出。患者啬啬恶寒,淅淅恶风,翕翕发热,另有鼻息鸣响和干呕等症状的,可用桂枝汤治疗。

Differentiation of pulse and syndrome / pattern [related to] taiyang disease and treatment (part 1)

fresh ginger, Rhizoma Zingiberis Recens) (cut) and 12 pieces of Dazao (大枣, jujube, Fructus Ziziphus Jujubae) (broken).

These five ingredients, [among which] three are broken into small pieces, [are decocted in] 7 *sheng* of water with mild fire till 3 *sheng* left [after boiling]. The dregs are removed and [the decoction is] taken warm 1 *sheng* [each time]. [After] taking the decoction [for a while], [the patient should] take 1 *sheng* of hot porridge to improve the effect of the decoction. [The patient can put on more clothes or cover himself with thick quilt in order to] warm the body and mildly promote sweating [for the purpose of] healing [the disease]. [But] sweating cannot be profuse, [otherwise] the disease is hard to heal. If the disease is cured through sweating [after] taking [the first *sheng* of decoction], [there is] no need to take [the decoction again and it is certainly] unnecessary to take all the decoction. If [there is] no sweating [after taking the first *sheng* of decoction, it is necessary] to take [the decoction] again according to the previous way. [If there is] no sweating [after taking the second *sheng* of the decoction], the rest [of the decoction should be] taken within half a day. If the disease is severe, [the decoction should be] taken day and night with careful observation all the time. [If] the disease is not eliminated [after] taking the first dose [of the decoction], [it should be] taken again. If sweating is absent, [the patient can] take two or three doses [of the decoction]. [When taking the decoction, the following foods and vegetables should be] prohibited, raw and cold foods, sticky and slimy foods, noodles cooked with meat, five kinds of acrid foods (including garlic, rocambole, semen brassicae campestris, coriander and animal milk) and wine, cheese and foods with special taste.

【原文】

(一三)

太阳病,头痛,发热,汗出,恶风,桂枝汤主之。

【今译】

太阳病,患者有头痛、发热、出汗、畏风症状的,用桂枝汤主治。

【原文】

(一四)

太阳病,项背强几几,反汗出恶风者,桂枝加葛根汤主之。

桂枝加葛根汤方

葛根四两、麻黄三两(去节)、芍药二两、生姜三两(切)、甘草二两(炙)、大枣十二枚(擘)、桂枝二两(去皮)。

右七味,以水一斗,先煮麻黄、葛根,减二升,去上沫,内诸药,煮取三升,去滓,温服一升,复取微似汗,不须啜粥,余如桂枝法将息及禁忌。

【今译】

太阳病,患者项部连背部强直,反而出汗恶风,用桂枝加葛根汤主治。

Differentiation of pulse and syndrome/pattern [related to] taiyang disease and treatment（part 1）

【英译】

Line 13

Taiyang disease [characterized by] headache，fever，sweating and aversion to wind can be treated by Guizhi Decoction（桂枝汤，cinnamon twig decoction）.

【英译】

Line 14

Taiyang disease [characterized by] stiffness of nape and back，sweating and aversion to wind can be treated by Guizhi Decoction（桂枝汤，cinnamon twig decoction）added with Gegen（葛根，pueraria，Radix Puerariae）.

Guizhi Decoction（桂枝汤，cinnamon twig decoction）added with Gegen（葛根，pueraria，Radix Puerariae Lobate）[is composed of] 4 *liang* of Gegen（葛根，pueraria，Radix Puerariae Lobate），3 *liang* of Mahuang（麻黄，ephedra，Herba Ephedrae）（nodes-removed），2 *liang* of Shaoyao（芍药，peony，Radix Paeoniae），3 *liang* of Shengjiang（生姜，fresh ginger，Rhizoma Zingiberis Recens）（cut），2 *liang* of Gancao（甘草，licorice，Radix Glycyrrhizae Praeparata）（broiled），12 pieces of Dazao（大枣，jujube，Fructus Ziziphus Jujubae）（broken）and 2 *liang* of Guizhi（桂枝，cinnamon twig，Ramulus Cinnamomi）（peel-removed）.

These seven ingredients are decocted in 1 *dou* of water. Mahuang（麻黄，ephedra，Herba Ephedrae）and Gegen（葛根，pueraria，Radix Puerariae Lobate）are decocted first till 8 *sheng* of water left. The foam is removed and other ingredients are put into [it to decoct till] 3 *sheng* of water left. The dregs are removed and [the decoction is] taken warm 1 *sheng* [each time]. [Then the patient is] covered [with quilt or clothes to] induce light sweating. [There is] no need to take porridge [after taking the deocction]. Contraindications are the same as that for Guizhi Decoction（桂枝汤，cinnamon twig decoction）.

【原文】

(一五)

太阳病,下之后,其气上冲者,可与桂枝汤,方用前法;若不上冲者,不得与之。

【今译】

太阳病,泻下之后,胸中有气逆上冲,可以用桂枝汤治疗,服药方法同前。若误下后没有气逆上冲的,则不能用桂枝汤治疗。

【原文】

(一六)

太阳病三日,已发汗,若吐、若下、若温针,仍不解者,此为坏病,桂枝不中与之也,观其脉证,知犯何逆,随证治之。桂枝本为解肌,若其人脉浮紧,发热汗不出者,不可与之也。常须识此,勿令误也。

【今译】

太阳病三日,已用过发汗法治疗,如果再用涌吐,或攻下,或温针等方法治疗,而病仍不解的,是因治疗不当而造成的坏病,桂枝汤不宜使用。观察脉症的变化,了解如何造成的逆变,随症选择治法。桂枝汤本来是用以解肌的,如果患者的脉象浮紧,发热而不出汗的,不可用桂枝汤治疗,应牢记桂枝汤的作用,不要误用。

Differentiation of pulse and syndrome/pattern [related to] taiyang disease and treatment (part 1)

【英译】

Line 15

Taiyang disease with up-flow of qi after purgation can be treated by Guizhi Decoction (桂枝汤，cinnamon twig decoction) as used previously. If there is no up-flow [of qi], [Guizhi Decoction (桂枝汤，cinnamon twig decoction)] cannot be used.

【英译】

Line 16

Taiyang disease with sweating [that has already been treated by] either vomiting, or purgation or [acupuncture with] warmed needle but is still not relieved, it is a severe disease and cannot be treated by Guizhi Decoction (桂枝汤，cinnamon twig decoction). Examination of the pulse can reveal its adverseness [and can make it clear about how to] treat such a syndrome/pattern. Guizhi Decoction (桂枝汤，cinnamon twig decoction) is usually used to relieve muscles. If the pulse is floating and tight and there is fever without sweating, [Guizhi Decoction (桂枝汤，cinnamon twig decoction)] cannot be used. [Such a caution must be] always borne in mind to avoid any mistreatment.

【原文】

(一七)

若酒客病,不可与桂枝汤,得之则呕,以酒客不喜甘故也。

【今译】

嗜酒患者,不可用桂枝汤治疗,若服用了桂枝汤,就会出现呕吐症状,这是因为嗜酒人不喜欢甘味的缘故。

【原文】

(一八)

喘家作桂枝汤,加厚朴、杏子佳。

桂枝三两(去皮)、甘草二两(炙)、生姜三两(切)、芍药三两、大枣十二枚(擘)、厚朴二两(炙,去皮)、杏仁五十枚(去皮尖)。

右七味,以水七升,微火煮取三升,去滓,温服一升,覆取微似汗。

【今译】

素有喘病的患者,桂枝汤加厚朴、杏仁治疗,效果更佳。

Differentiation of pulse and syndrome / pattern [related to] taiyang disease and treatment（part 1）

【英译】

Line 17

Disease［caused by addict to］drinking wine cannot be treated by Guizhi Decoction（桂枝汤，cinnamon twig decoction）［which may］cause vomiting because the patient with alcoholism does not like sweet taste.

【英译】

Line 18

The patient［suffering from］asthma can be treated by Guizhi Decoction（桂枝汤，cinnamon twig decoction）added with Houpo（厚朴，magnolia bark，Cortex Magnoliae Officinalis）and Xingren（杏仁，apricot kernel，Semen Armeniacae Amarum）.

Guizhi Decoction（桂枝汤，cinnamon twig decoction）added with Houpo（厚朴，magnolia bark，Cortex Magnoliae Officinalis）and Xingren（杏仁，apricot kernel，Semen Armeniacae Amarum）［is composed of］3 *liang* of Guizhi（桂枝，cinnamon twig，Ramulus Cinnamomi）(bark-removed)，2 *liang* of Gancao（甘草，licorice，Radix Glycyrrhizae Praeparata）(broiled)，3 *liang* of Shengjiang（生姜，fresh ginger，Rhizoma Zingiberis Recens）(cut)，3 *liang* of Shaoyao（芍药，peony，Radix Paeoniae），12 pieces of Dazao（大枣，jujube，Fructus Ziziphus Jujubae）(broken)，2 *liang* of Houpo（厚朴，magnolia bark，Cortex Magnoliae Officinalis）(broiled and peel-removed) and 50 pieces of Xingren（杏仁，apricot kernel，Semen Armeniacae Amarum）(peel-and-tips-removed).

These seven ingredients are decocted in 7 *sheng* of water in mild fire to get 3 *sheng*［after］boiling. The dregs are removed and［the decoction］is taken warm 1 *sheng*［each time］.［Then the patient is］covered［with quilt or clothes to］induce light sweating.

【原文】

(一九)

凡服桂枝汤吐者,其后必吐脓血也。

【今译】

凡服用桂枝汤而发生呕吐的,以后可能会出现吐脓血的变症。

【原文】

(二〇)

太阳病,发汗,遂漏不止,其人恶风,小便难,四肢微急,难以屈伸者,桂枝加附子汤主之。

桂枝加附子汤方

桂枝三两(去皮)、芍药三两、甘草三两(炙)、生姜三两(切)、大枣十二枚(擘)、附子一枚(炮,去皮,破八片)。

右六味,以水七升,煮取三升,去滓,温服一升。本云桂枝汤,今加附子,将息如前法。

【今译】

太阳病,发汗太过可致汗出淋漓不止、病人恶风、小便不畅、四肢略微拘急、屈伸困难,用桂枝加附子汤主治。

Differentiation of pulse and syndrome/pattern [related to] taiyang disease and treatment (part 1)

【英译】

Line 19

[The patient who] vomits after taking Guizhi Decoction (桂枝汤, cinnamon decoction) will inevitably vomit bloody pus.

【英译】

Line 20

[The patient with] taiyang disease perspires severely like leaking water [after treatment with] diaphoresis, [indicating that there are symptoms of] aversion to wind, difficulty in defecation, slight stiffness of the four limbs difficult to bend and extend, [which can be] treated by Guizhi Decoction (桂枝汤, cinnamon twig decoction) added with Fuzi (附子, aconite, Radix Aconiti Lateralis Preparata).

Guizhi Decoction (桂枝汤, cinnamon twig decoction) added with Fuzi (附子, aconite, Radix Aconiti Lateralis Preparata) [is composed of] 3 *liang* of Guizhi (桂枝, cinnamon twig, Ramulus Cinnamomi) (bark-removed), 3 *liang* of Shaoyao (芍药, peony, Radix Paeoniae), 3 *liang* of Gancao (甘草, licorice, Radix Glycyrrhizae Praeparata) (broiled), 3 *liang* of Shengjiang (生姜, fresh ginger, Rhizoma Zingiberis Recens)(cut), 12 pieces of Dazao (大枣, jujube, Fructus Ziziphus Jujubae) (broken) and 1 piece of Fuzi (附子, aconite, Radix Aconiti Lateralis Preparata) (fried heavily, peel-removed, pound into eight small pieces).

These six ingredients are decocted in 7 *sheng* of water to get 3 *sheng* [after] boiling. The dregs are removed and [the decoction is] taken warm 1 *sheng* [each time]. The old edition says that Guizhi Decoction (桂枝汤, cinnamon twig decoction) added with Fuzi (附子, aconite, Radix Aconiti Lateralis Preparata) is used in the same way [of Guizhi Decoction (桂枝汤, cinnamon twig decoction)].

【原文】

（二一）

太阳病，下之后，脉促胸满者，桂枝去芍药汤主之。

桂枝去芍药汤方

桂枝三两（去皮）、甘草二两（炙）、生姜三两（切）、大枣十二枚（擘）。

右四味，以水七升，煮取三升，去滓，温服一升。本云桂枝汤，今去芍药，将息如前法。

【今译】

太阳病，攻下之后，出现脉象急促、胸部胀闷等症状的，用桂枝去芍药汤主治。

Differentiation of pulse and syndrome / pattern [related to] taiyang disease and treatment (part 1)

【英译】

Line 21

Taiyang disease with rapid pulse and chest fullness [can be] treated by Guizhi Decoction (桂枝汤, cinnamon twig decoction) without Shaoyao (芍药, peony, Radix Paeoniae).

Guizhi Decoction (桂枝汤, cinnamon twig decoction) without Shaoyao (芍药, peony, Radix Paeoniae) [is composed of] 3 *liang* of Guizhi (桂枝, cinnamon twig, Ramulus Cinnamomi) (bark-removed), 2 *liang* of Gancao (甘草, licorice, Radix Glycyrrhizae Praeparata) (broiled), 3 *liang* of Shengjiang (生姜, fresh ginger, Rhizoma Zingiberis Recens) (cut) and 12 pieces of Dazao (大枣, jujube, Fructus Ziziphus Jujubae) (broken).

These four ingredients are decocted in 7 *sheng* of water to get 3 *sheng* [after] boiling. The dregs are removed and [the decoction is] taken warm 1 *sheng* [each time]. The old edition says that Guizhi Decoction (桂枝汤, cinnamon twig decoction) without Shaoyao (芍药, peony, Radix Paeoniae) is used in the same way [of Guizhi Decoction (桂枝汤, cinnamon twig decoction)].

【原文】

（二二）

若微寒者,桂枝去芍药加附子汤主之。

桂枝去芍药加附子汤方

桂枝三两(去皮)、甘草二两(炙)、生姜三两(切)、大枣十二枚(擘)

附子一枚(炮,去皮,破八片)。

右五味,以水七升,煮取三升,去滓,温服一升。本云桂枝汤,今去

芍药加附子,将息如前法。

【今译】

若患者有微寒症状,用桂枝去芍药加附子汤主治。

Differentiation of pulse and syndrome / pattern
[related to] taiyang disease and treatment (part 1)

【英译】

Line 22

[The patient with] slight cold [can be] treated by Guizhi Decoction（桂枝汤，cinnamon twig decoction）with Shaoyao（芍药，peony，Radix Paeoniae）removed and Fuzi（附子，aconite，Radix Aconiti Lateralis Preparata）added.

Guizhi Decoction（桂枝汤，cinnamon twig decoction）with Shaoyao（芍药，peony，Radix Paeoniae）removed and Fuzi（附子，aconite，Radix Aconiti Lateralis Preparata）added [is composed of] 3 *liang* of Guizhi（桂枝，cinnamon twig，Ramulus Cinnamomi）（bark-removed），2 *liang* of Gancao（甘草，licorice，Radix Glycyrrhizae Praeparata）（broiled），3 *liang* of Shengjiang（生姜，fresh ginger，Rhizoma Zingiberis Recens）（cut），12 pieces of Dazao（大枣，jujube，Fructus Ziziphus Jujubae）（broken）and 1 piece of Fuzi（附子，aconite，Radix Aconiti Lateralis Preparata）（fried heavily，peel-removed，pound into eight small pieces）.

These five ingredients are decocted in 7 *sheng* of water to get 3 *sheng* [after] boiling. The dregs are removed and [the decoction is] taken warm 1 *sheng* [each time]. The old edition says that Guizhi Decoction（桂枝汤，cinnamon twig decoction）with Shaoyao（芍药，peony，Radix Paeoniae）removed and Fuzi（附子，aconite，Radix Aconiti Lateralis Preparata）added is used in the same way [of Guizhi Decoction（桂枝汤，cinnamon twig decoction）].

【原文】

(二三)

太阳病,得之八九日,如疟状,发热恶寒,热多寒少,其人不呕,清便欲自可,一日二三度发。脉微缓者,为欲愈也;脉微而恶寒者,此阴阳俱虚,不可更发汗、更下、更吐也;面色反有热色者,未欲解也,以其不能得小汗出,身必痒,宜桂枝麻黄各半汤。

桂枝麻黄各半汤方

桂枝一两十六铢(去皮),芍药、生姜(切)、甘草(炙)、麻黄各一两(去节),大枣四枚(擘),杏仁二十四枚(汤浸,去皮尖及两仁者)。

右七味,以水五升,先煮麻黄一两沸,去上沫,内诸药,煮取一升八合,去滓,温服六合。本云桂枝汤三合,麻黄汤三合,并为六合,顿服,将息如上法。

【今译】

太阳病发作八九天后,其发热恶寒,形似疟疾,发热时间长,恶寒时间短,患者不呕吐,大小便正常,每日发作两三次。如果脉象微缓,即为将要痊愈的表现。如果脉象微而恶寒,表明阴阳俱虚,不可再使用发汗、攻下或涌吐之法治疗。如果患者面部出现热红色,说明表证并未解除,因此也没有微汗出现,而患者的身心必有发痒的感觉。对于这样的病变,可采用桂枝麻黄各半汤治疗。

Differentiation of pulse and syndrome/pattern [related to] taiyang disease and treatment (part 1)

【英译】

Line 23

[In] Taiyang disease, eight or nine days after occurrence, [the symptoms] like malaria, fever, aversion to cold, severe heat and slight cold, no vomiting, normal urination and defecation, may occur two or three times a day. [If] the pulse is slight and slow, [it] will heal. [If] the pulse is slight and [there is] aversion to cold, [it indicates] dual deficiency of yin and yang, [which] cannot be treated further by [the therapies for] diaphoresis, purgation and vomiting. [If] the facial complexion appears feverish, [it cannot] heal right now due to no slight sweating [that causes] itching of the body. [Such a case can be] treated by the Decoction composed of half of Guizhi Decoction (桂枝汤, cinnamon twig decoction) and half of Mahuang Decoction (麻黄汤, ephedra decoction).

This formula [is composed of] 1 *liang* and 16 *zhu* of Guizhi (桂枝, cinnamon twig, Ramulus Cinnamomi) (bark-removed), 1 *liang* of Shaoyao (芍药, peony, Radix Paeoniae), 1 *liang* of Shengjiang (生姜, fresh ginger, Rhizoma Zingiberis Recens)(cut), 1 *liang* of Gancao (甘草, licorice, Radix Glycyrrhizae Praeparata) (broiled), 1 *liang* of Mahuang (麻黄, ephedra, Herba Ephedrae) (node-removed), 4 pieces of Dazao (大枣, jujube, Fructus Ziziphus Jujubae) (broken)and 24 pieces of Fuzi (附子, aconite, Radix Aconiti Lateralis Preparata) (soaked in the decoction).

These seven ingredients are decocted 5 *sheng* of water. Mahuang (Herba Ephedrae) is decocted first for once or twice. The foam is removed and other ingredients are put into [it to decoct and get] 1 *sheng* and 8 *ge* of water [after] boiling. The dregs are removed and [the decoction is] taken warm 6 *ge* [each time]. The old edition says that 3 *ge* of Guizhi Decoction (桂枝汤, cinnamon twig decoction) is combined with 3 *ge* of Mahuang Decoction (麻黄汤, ephedra decoction), altogether 6 *ge* [which is] taken all the whole for once. [This decoction] is used in the same way [of Guizhi Decoction (桂枝汤, cinnamon twig decoction].

【原文】

(二四)

太阳病,初服桂枝汤,反烦不解者,先刺风池、风府,却与桂枝汤则愈。

【今译】

太阳病,初次服用桂枝汤后,反而引起烦闷不解,可先刺风池、风府穴,然后用桂枝汤,就能痊愈。

【原文】

(二五)

服桂枝汤,大汗出,脉洪大者,与桂枝汤,如前法。若形似疟,一日再发者,汗出必解,宜桂枝二麻黄一汤。

桂枝二麻黄一汤方

桂枝一两十七铢(去皮)、芍药一两六铢、麻黄十六铢(去节)、生姜一两六铢(切)、杏仁十六个(去皮尖)、甘草一两三铢(炙)、大枣五枚(擘)。

右七味,以水五升,先煮麻黄一二沸,去上沫,内诸药,煮取二升,去滓,温服一升,日再服。本云桂枝汤二分,麻黄汤一分,合为二升,分再服,今合为一方,将息如前法。

Differentiation of pulse and syndrome / pattern ⌈related to⌉ taiyang disease and treatment（part 1）

【英译】

Line 24

⌈If⌉ Taiyang disease is first treated by Guizhi Decoction（桂枝汤，cinnamon twig decoction）but fails to heal and ⌈makes the patient feel⌉ listless，⌈it can be treated⌉ first by needling Fengchi（GB 21）and Fengfu（GV 16）and then by Guizhi Decoction（桂枝汤，cinnamon twig decoction）.

【英译】

Line 25

⌈If the patient⌉ perspires heavily and the pulse is full and large ⌈after⌉ taking Guizhi Decoction（桂枝汤，cinnamon twig decoction），it still can be used as applied previously. If it appears like malaria and recurs one day after，diaphoresis must be used，and the Decoction ⌈containing⌉ two Guizhi Decoction（桂枝汤，cinnamon twig decoction）and one Mahuang Decoction（麻黄汤，ephedra decoction）is also necessary.

This formula ⌈is composed of⌉ 1 *liang* and 17 *zhu* of Guizhi（桂枝，cinnamon twig，Ramulus Cinnamomi）（bark-removed），1 *liang* and 6 *zhu* of Shaoyao（芍药，peony，Radix Paeoniae），16 *zhu* of Mahuang（麻黄，ephedra，Herba Ephedrae）（nodes-removed），1 *liang* and 6 *zhu* of Shengjiang（生姜，fresh ginger，Rhizoma Zingiberis Recens）（cut），16 pieces of Xingren（杏仁，apricot kernel，Semen Armeniacae Amarum）（peel-and-tips-removed），1 and 3 *zhu* of Gancao（甘草，licorice，Radix Glycyrrhizae Praeparata）（broiled）and 5 pieces of Dazao（大枣，jujube，Fructus Ziziphus Jujubae）（broken）.

These seven ingredients are decocted in 5 *sheng* of water. Mahuang（麻黄，ephedra，Herba Ephedrae）is decocted first for once or twice. The foam is removed and other ingredients are put into ⌈it to decoct and get⌉ 2 *sheng* ⌈after⌉ boiling. The dregs are

【今译】

　　服用桂枝汤后,引起大出汗,脉洪大的,仍用桂枝汤治疗,方法如前所述。若症状像疟疾,第二天再次发作,以发汗法治之必能解除。可用桂枝二麻黄一汤主治。

【原文】

　　(二六)

　　服桂枝汤,大汗出后,大烦渴不解,脉洪大者,白虎加人参汤主之。

　　白虎加人参汤方

　　知母六两、石膏一斤(碎,绵裹)、甘草二两(炙)、粳米六合、人参三两。

　　右五味,以水一斗,煮米熟汤成,去滓,温服一升,日三服。

【今译】

　　患者服用桂枝汤后,大汗已出,但大烦渴却不解,脉象洪大的,用白虎加人参汤主治。

Differentiation of pulse and syndrome / pattern [related to] taiyang disease and treatment (part 1)

removed and [the decoction is] taken warm 1 *sheng* [each time] and twice a day. The old edition says that 2 *fen* of Guizhi Decoction (桂枝汤，cinnamon twig decoction) is combined with 1 *fen* of Mahuang Decoction (麻黄汤，ephedra decoction)，and altogether there is 2 *sheng* [which is] taken [1 *sheng* each time and] twice a day. This combined decoction is used in the same way [of Guizhi Decoction (桂枝汤，cinnamon twig decoction)].

【英译】

Line 26

[After] taking Guizhi Decoction （桂枝汤，cinnamon twig decoction）and profuse sweating，[if the patient feels] restless and thirsty with full and large pulse，[it can be] treated by Baihu Decoction （白虎汤，white tiger decoction）added with Renshen （人参，ginseng，Radix Ginseng）.

Baihu Decoction （白虎汤，white tiger decoction）added with Renshen （人参，ginseng，Radix Ginseng）[is composed of] 6 *liang* of Zhimu （知母，anemarrhena，Rhizoma Anemarrhenae），1 *jin* of Shigao （石膏，gypsum，Gypsum Fibrosum）to be broken into small pieces and kept in a cotton gauze，2 *liang* of Gancao （甘草，licorice，Radix Glycyrrhizae Praeparata）（broiled），6 *ge* of Jingmi （粳米，polished round-grained rice，Semen Oryzae Nonglutinosae）and 3 *liang* of Renshen （人参，ginseng，Radix Ginseng）.

These five ingredients are decocted in 1 *dou* of water till Jingmi （粳米，polished round-grained rice，Semen Oryzae Sativae）is well cooked. The dregs are removed and [the decoction is] taken warm 1 *sheng* [each time] and three times a day.

【原文】

（二七）

太阳病，发热恶寒，热多寒少，脉微弱者，此无阳也，不可发汗，宜桂枝二越婢一汤。

桂枝二越婢一汤方

桂枝（去皮），芍药、麻黄、甘草各十八铢（炙），大枣四枚（擘），生姜一两三钱（切），石膏二十四铢（碎，绵裹）。

右七味，以水五升，煮麻黄一两沸，去上沫，内诸药，煮取二升，去滓，温服一升。本云：当裁为越婢汤桂枝汤合之饮一升，今合为一方，桂枝汤二分，越婢汤一分。

【今译】

太阳病患者，有发热恶寒，发热时间长，恶寒时间短，脉象微弱等症状，此无阳也，不可发汗，可用桂枝二越婢一汤治疗。

Differentiation of pulse and syndrome / pattern [related to] taiyang disease and treatment (part 1)

【英译】

Line 27

Taiyang disease，[with the symptoms and signs of] fever，aversion to cold，more heat and less cold，slight and weak pulse，[indicates that there is] no yang and diaphoresis cannot be used．[Only the Decoction composed of] two Guizhi Decoction（桂枝汤，cinnamon twig decoction）and one Yuebi Decoction（越婢汤，decoction for effusing the spleen）can be used．

This formula [is composed of] 18 *zhu* of Guizhi（桂枝，cinnamon twig，Ramulus Cinnamomi）with bark removed，18 *zhu* of Shaoyao（芍药，peony，Radix Paeoniae），18 *zhu* of Mahuang（麻黄，ephedra，Radix Ephedrae），18 *zhu* of Gancao（甘草，licorice，Radix Glycyrrhizae Praeparata）（broiled），4 pieces of Dazao（大枣，jujube，Fructus Ziziphus Jujubae）（broken），1 *liang* and 3 *zhu* of Shengjiang（生姜，fresh ginger，Rhizoma Zingiberis Recens）（cut）and 24 *zhu* of Shigao（石膏，gysum，Gypsum Fibrosum）（pound，wrapped in a cotton gauze）．

These seven ingredients are decocted in 5 *sheng* of water． Mahuang（麻黄，ephedra，Herba Ephedrae）is decocted first for once or twice．The foam is removed and other ingredients are put into [it to decoct and get] 2 *sheng* [after] boiling．The dregs are removed and [the decoction is] taken warm 1 *sheng* [each time]． The old edition says that this decoction is a combination of Yuebi Decoction（越婢汤，decoction for effusing the spleen）and Guizhi Decoction（桂枝汤，cinnamon twig decoction）and [should be] taken 1 *sheng* [each time]．Now [these two decoctions are] combined into one [which is]composed of 2 tenth of Guizhi Decoction（桂枝汤，cinnamon twig decoction）and 1 tenth of Yuebi Decoction（越婢汤，decoction for effusing the spleen）．

【原文】

(二八)

服桂枝汤,或下之,仍头项强痛,翕翕发热,无汗,心下满微痛,小便不利者,桂枝去桂加茯苓白术汤主之。

桂枝去桂加茯苓白术汤方

芍药三两,甘草二两(炙)、生姜(切)、白术、茯苓各三两,大枣十二枚。

右六味,以水八升,煮取三升,取滓,温服一升,小便利则愈。本云桂枝汤,今去桂枝,加茯苓、白术。

【今译】

服用了桂枝汤,或使用了泻下法,但患者却仍然头部和项部强痛,身上翕翕发热,无汗,心下胀满,微感疼痛,小便不畅,可用桂枝汤去桂枝加茯苓白术汤治疗。

Differentiation of pulse and syndrome／pattern ［related to］ taiyang disease and treatment（part 1）

【英译】

Line 28

［After］ taking Guizhi Decoction（桂枝汤，cinnamon twig decoction）or ［treated by］ purgation，［there are］ still ［symptoms and signs of］ stiffness and pain of head and nape，constant fever，no sweating，abdominal fullness，slight pain and dysuria，［it can be］ treated by Guizhi Decoction（桂枝汤，cinnamon twig decoction）with Fuling（茯苓，poria，Poria）and Baizhu（白术，Largehead Atractylodes Rhizome，Rhizoma Atractylodis Macrocephalae）added and Guizhi（桂枝，Ramulus Cinnamomi）removed.

Guizhi Decoction（桂枝汤，cinnamon twig decoction）with Fuling（茯苓，poria，Poria）and Baizhu（白术，Largehead Atractylodes Rhizome，Rhizoma Atractylodis Macrocephalae）added and Guizhi（Ramulus Cinnamomi）removed ［is composed of］ 3 *liang* of Shaoyao（芍药，peony，Radix Paeoniae），2 *liang* of Gancao（甘草，licorice，Radix Glycyrrhizae Praeparata）（broiled），3 *liang* of Shengjiang（生姜，fresh ginger，Rhizoma Zingiberis Recens）（cut），3 *liang* of Baizhu（白术，Largehead Atractylodes Rhizome，Rhizoma Atractylodis Macrocephalae），3 *liang* of Fuling（茯苓，poria，Poria）and 12 pieces of Dazao（大枣，jujube，Fructus Ziziphus Jujubae）.

These six ingredients are decocted in 8 *sheng* of water to get 3 *sheng* ［after］boiling. The dregs are removed and ［the decoction is］ taken warm 1 *sheng* ［each time］. ［When］ urination is normalized，［the disease will］ heal. The old edition says that Guizhi Decoction（桂枝汤，cinnamon twig decoction）［should be used］. Now Guizhi（桂枝，cinnamon twig，Ramulus Cinnamomi）is removed ［while］ Fuling（茯苓，poria，Poria）and Baizhu（白术，Largehead Atractylodes Rhizome，Rhizoma Atractylodis Macrocephalae）are added.

【原文】

(二九)

伤寒,脉浮,自汗出,小便数,心烦,微恶寒,脚挛急,反与桂枝欲攻其表,此误也。得之便厥,咽中干,烦躁吐逆者,作甘草干姜汤与之,以复其阳。若厥愈足温者,更作芍药甘草汤与之,其脚即伸。若胃气不和,谵语者,少与调胃承气汤。若重发汗,复加烧针者,四逆汤主之。

甘草干姜汤方

甘草四两(炙)、干姜二两。

右二味,以水三升,煮取一升五合,去滓,分温再服。

芍药甘草汤方

白芍药、甘草各四两(炙)。

右二味,以水三升,煮取一升五合,去滓,分温再服。

调胃承气汤方

大黄四两,去皮。用陈米酒洗甘草二两,炙芒硝半升。

右三味,以水三升,煮取一升,去滓,内芒硝,更上火,微煮令沸,少少温服之。

四逆汤方

甘草二两,炙干姜一两半,附子一枚,用生,去皮,破成八片。

Differentiation of pulse and syndrome / pattern
[related to] taiyang disease and treatment (part 1)

【英译】

Line 29

Cold damage [characterized by] floating pulse, spontaneous sweating, frequent urination, dysphoria, slight aversion to cold and spasm of feet seems to be attacked of the superficies after taking Guizhi Decoction (桂枝汤, cinnamon twig decoction). This is a wrong treatment [which will] cause reversal [cold of limbs]. [The patient with] dry throat, dysphoria, vomiting and nausea can be treated by Gancao Ganjiang Decoction (甘草干姜汤, licorice and dried ginger decoction) to restore yang. When cold is relieved and the feet are warmed up, Shaoyao Gancao Decoction (芍药甘草汤, peony and licorice decoction) can be used to relieve spasm of foot. If [there are symptoms and signs of] disharmony of stomach qi and delirium, Tiaowei Chengqi Decoction (调胃承气汤, decoction for regulating the stomach and harmonizing qi) can be used in small dosage. If [there is] heavy sweating already treated by acupuncture with heated needle, [it can be] treated by Sini Decoction (四逆汤, decoction for resolving four kinds of adverseness).

Gancao Ganjiang Decoction (甘草干姜汤, licorice and dried ginger decoction) [is composed of] 4 *liang* of Gancao (甘草, licorice, Radix Glycyrrhizae) (broiled) and 2 *liang* of Ganjiang (干姜, dried ginger, Rhizoma Zingiberis).

These two ingredients are decocted in 3 *sheng* of water to get 1. 5 *sheng* [after] boiling. After dregs removed, the decoction can be divided into two doses and taken warm.

Shaoyao Gancao Decoction (芍药甘草汤, peony and licorice decoction) [is composed of] 4 *liang* of Shaoyao (芍药, peony,

右三味,以水三升,煮取一升二合,去滓,分温再服。强人可大附子一枚,干姜三两。

【今译】

伤寒病,出现脉浮、汗自出、小便频数、心烦、轻微恶寒、腿脚拘急,若用桂枝汤解表,是错误治法。服药后就会出现四肢冰冷、咽喉干燥、烦躁不安、呕吐等症状,可先用甘草干姜汤,使阳气复来。服了甘草干姜汤后,四肢由厥冷转愈为腿足温暖的,再用芍药甘草汤治疗,腿足即可伸展。如果患者胃气不和,且有谵语的,用少量调胃承气汤治疗。如果又反复发汗,再用烧针治疗,以四逆汤为主治。

Differentiation of pulse and syndrome / pattern [related to] taiyang disease and treatment (part 1)

Radix Paeoniae) and 4 *liang* of Gancao（甘草，licorice，Radix Glycyrrhizae Praeparata)（broiled）.

These two ingredients are decocted in 3 *sheng* of water to get 1.5 *sheng* [after] boiling. After dregs removed, the decoction can be divided into two doses and taken warm.

Tiaowei Chengqi Decoction （调胃承气汤，decoction for regulating the stomach and harmonizing qi）[is composed of] 4 *liang* of Dahuang（大黄，rhubarb，Radix et Rhizoma Rhei)（peel-removed），2 *liang* of Gancao（甘草，licorice，Radix Glycyrrhizae Praeparata)（washed in old rice wine)and 0.5 *sheng* of Mangxiao （芒硝，mirabilite，Natrii Sulfas)（broiled）.

These three medicinals are decocted in 3 *sheng* of water to get 1 *sheng* [after] boiling. After removal of dregs, Mangxiao（芒硝，mirabilite，Natrii Sulfas) is added to the decoction which is stewed again and boiled. Such a decoction can be taken warm once a little.

Sini Decoction（四逆汤，decoction for resolving four kinds of adverseness）[is composed of] 2 *liang* of Gancao（甘草，licorice，Radix Glycyrrhizae Praeparata），1.5 *liang* of Ganjiang（干姜，dried ginger，Rhizoma Zingiberis)（broiled) and 1 piece of Fuzi（附子，aconite，Radix Aconiti)（fresh，remove bark and break into 8 small pieces）.

These three ingredients are decocted in 3 *sheng* of water to get 1 *sheng* and 2 *ge* [after] boiling. The dregs are removed and [the decoction is] divided [into two doses] and taken warm. [For those who are] strong, 1 piece of big Fuzi（附子，aconite，Radix Aconiti) and 3 *liang* of Ganjiang（干姜，dried ginger，Rhizoma Zingiberis) can be used.

【原文】

(三〇)

问曰：证象阳旦，按法治之而增剧，厥逆，咽中干，两胫拘急而谵语。师曰：言夜半手足当温，两脚当伸。后如师言，何以知此？

答曰：寸口脉浮而大，浮为风，大为虚，风则生微热，虚则两胫挛，病形象桂枝，因加附子参其间。增桂令汗出，附子温经，亡阳故也。厥逆，咽中干，烦躁，阳明内结，谵语，烦乱，更饮甘草干姜汤。夜半阳气还，两足当热；胫尚微拘急，重与芍药甘草汤，尔乃胫伸。以承气汤微溏，则止其谵语，故知病可愈。

【今译】

问：患者的症状似桂枝汤证，按照其治法进行治疗，反而使病情加剧，出现四肢冰冷、咽喉干燥、两小腿肌肉拘急、谵语等症状。老师说患者半夜手足应当温暖，两腿应当能伸展。病情的发展果然如老师所说的那样，这是如何知道的呢？

老师回答说：病人寸口脉浮而大，脉浮体现的是风邪，脉大体现的是虚弱。风邪会引起轻微发热，虚弱则会出现小腿肌肉拘挛。症状像桂枝汤症，所以治疗上必须用桂枝汤加附子。如果单用桂枝汤发汗，会导致汗出亡阳，引起四肢冰冷、咽喉干燥、阳明内结、谵语、烦躁等症状。治疗时先用甘草干姜汤，服用后阳气于半夜恢复，两腿变温暖。但小腿肌肉拘挛尚未解除，可再用芍药甘草汤。服药后，两腿可自由伸展。用承气汤攻下后，大便微见溏泻，谵语等症则会停止，病即可痊愈。

Differentiation of pulse and syndrome/pattern [related to] taiyang disease and treatment (part 1)

【英译】

Line 30

Question: The syndrome/pattern appears like [the one to be treated by] Guizhi Decoction (桂枝汤, cinnamon twig decoction). [But when] treated by [Guizhi Decoction (桂枝汤, cinnamon twig decoction) it] becomes severe, [marked by] reversal cold [of limbs], dryness of throat, spasm of legs and delirium. Master has said [that the patient's] hands and feet will warm up in the midnight and the legs will be able to stretch. [What has happened] later on is just as [what] the master has said. What is the reason?

Answer: The cunkou pulse (wrist pulse) is floating and large. [Floating pulse] indicates wind [while] large [pulse] indicates deficiency. Wind causes slight heat [while] deficiency causes spasm of legs, the disease [caused by which is] similar to [the one to be treated by] Guizhi [Decoction (桂枝汤, cinnamon twig decoction)]. [To treat it with Guizhi Decoction (桂枝汤, cinnamon twig decoction),] Fuzi (附子, aconite, Radix Aconiti Lateralis Preparata) [should be] added. Addition [of Fuzi (附子, aconite, Radix Aconiti Lateralis Preparata)] to Guizhi [Decoction (桂枝汤, cinnamon twig decoction)] can induce sweating and warm meridians. [Just application of Guizhi Decoction (桂枝汤, cinnamon twig decoction) without addition of Fuzi (附子, aconite, Radix Aconiti Lateralis Preparata) will lead to] loss of yang [accompanied by] reversal cold [of limbs], dryness of throat, dysphoria, internal binding of yangming, delirium and restlessness, [which should be treated by] Gancao Ganjiang Decoction (甘草干姜汤, licorice and dried ginger decoction). [After treatment with such a decoction,] yang qi [will be] restored in the midnight, the feet [will certainly become] warm. [But] the legs are still spasmatic. [In this case] Shaoyao Gancao Decoction (芍药甘草汤, peony and licorice decoction) can be used [to disperse spasm] and [enable the legs to] stretch. [Then] Chengqi Decoction (承气汤, decoction for harmonizing qi) [can be used to induce] sloppy stool and cease delirium, and eventually healing the disease.

辨太阳病脉证并治中

【原文】

（三一）

太阳病，项背强几几，无汗，恶风，葛根汤主之。

葛根汤方

葛根四两、麻黄三两（去节）、桂枝二两（去皮）、芍药二两、生姜三两（切）、甘草二两（炙）、芍药二两、大枣十二枚（擘）。

右七味，以水一斗，先煮麻黄葛根，减二升，去白沫，内诸药，煮取三升，去滓，温服一升，复取微似汗，余如桂枝法将息及禁忌，诸汤皆仿此。

【今译】

太阳病，患者项背部拘紧，无汗，畏风，宜用葛根汤主治。

*Differentiation of pulse and syndrome / pattern
[related to] taiyang disease and treatment (part 2)*

Differentiation of pulse and syndrome/pattern [related to] taiyang disease and treatment (part 2)

【英译】

Line 31

Taiyang disease, [characterized by] stiffness of nape and back, no sweating and aversion to cold, [can be] treated by Gegen Decoction (葛根汤, pueraria decoction).

Gegen Decoction (葛根汤, pueraria decoction) [is composed of] 4 *liang* of Gegen (葛根, pueraria, Radix Puerariae), 3 *liang* of Mahuang (麻黄, ephedra, Herba Ephedrae) (node-removed), 2 *liang* of Guizhi (桂枝, cinnamon twig, Ramulus Cinnamomi) (bark-removed), 2 *liang* of Shaoyao (芍药, peony, Radix Paeoniae), 3 *liang* of Shengjiang (生姜, fresh ginger, Rhizoma Zingiberis Recens) (cut), 2 *liang* of Gancao (甘草, licorice, Radix Glycyrrhizae Praeparata) (broiled) and 12 pieces of Dazao (大枣, jujube, Fructus Ziziphus Jujubae) (broken).

These seven ingredients mentioned above [are decocted] in 1 *dou* of water to reduce 2 *sheng* of water. Mahuang (麻黄, ephedra, Herba Ephedrae) and Gegen (葛根, pueraria, Radix Puerariae) are decocted first. The foam is removed and other ingredients are put into [it to decoct and get] 3 *sheng* [after] boiling. The dregs are removed and [the decoction is] taken warm 1 *sheng* [each time]. [Then the patient is] covered [with quilt or clothes to] induce light sweating. Contraindications are the same as that for Guizhi (桂枝汤, cinnamon twig decoction), [which can be] followed by decoctions [of other categories].

【原文】

(三二)

太阳与阳明合病者,必自下利,葛根汤主之。

【今译】

太阳与阳明合病时,必然导致腹泻,宜用葛根汤主治。

【原文】

(三三)

太阳与阳明合病,不下利,但呕者,葛根加半夏汤主之。

葛根加半夏汤方

葛根四两、麻黄三两(去节)、甘草二两(炙)、芍药二两、桂枝二两(去皮)、生姜三两(切)、半夏半升(洗)、大枣十二枚(擘)。

右八味,以水一斗,先煮葛根、麻黄,减二升,去白沫,内诸药,煮取三升,去滓,温服一升,覆取微似汗。

【今译】

太阳与阳明合病时,患者没有腹泻,但作呕,宜用葛根加半夏汤主治。

Differentiation of pulse and syndrome/pattern [related to] taiyang disease and treatment (part 2)

【英译】

Line 32

Disease [due to invasion of pathogenic factors into] both taiyang [meridian] and yangming [meridian] causes diarrhea [and can be] treated by Gegen Decoction (葛根汤, pueraria decoction).

【英译】

Line 33

Disease [due to invasion of pathogenic factors into] both taiyang [meridian] and yangming [meridian] causes no diarrhea but vomiting [and can be] treated by Gegen Decoction (葛根汤, pueraria decoction) added with Banxia (半夏, pinellia, Rhizoma Pinelliae).

Gegen Decoction (葛根汤, pueraria decoction) added with Banxia (半夏, pinellia, Rhizoma Pinelliae) [is composed of] 4 *liang* of Gegen (葛根, pueraria, Radix Puerariae), 3 *liang* of Mahuang (麻黄, ephedra, Herba Ephedrae) (nodes-removed), 2 *liang* of Gancao (甘草, licorice, Radix Glycyrrhizae Praeparata) (broiled), 2 *liang* of Shaoyao (芍药, peony, Radix Paeoniae), 2 *liang* of Guizhi (桂枝, cinnamon twig, Ramulus Cinnamomi) (bark-removed), 3 *liang* of Shengjiang (生姜, fresh ginger, Rhizoma Zingiberis Recens) (cut), 0.5 *sheng* of Banxia (半夏, pinellia, Rhizoma Pinelliae) (wasked) and 12 pieces of Dazao (大枣, jujube, Fructus Ziziphus Jujubae) (broken).

These eight ingredients are decocted in 1 *dou* of water. Gegen (葛根, pueraria, Radix Puerariae) and Mahuang (麻黄, ephedra, Herba Ephedrae) are decocted first to reduce 2 *sheng* [of water]. The foam is removed and the rest medicinals are put into [it to decoct and to get] 3 *sheng* [after] boiling. The dregs are removed and [the decoction is] taken warm 1 *sheng* [each time]. [Then the patient is] covered [with quilt or clothes to] induce light sweating.

【原文】

(三四)

太阳病,桂枝证,医反下之,利遂不止,脉促者,表未解也。喘而汗出者,葛根黄芩黄连汤主之。

葛根黄芩黄连汤方

葛根半斤、甘草二两(炙)、黄芩二两、黄连三两。

右四味,以水八升,先煮葛根,减二升,内诸药,煮取二升,去滓,分温再服。

【今译】

太阳病,属桂枝汤证,本应用汗法,但医生却反而用下法,从而导致腹泻不止,脉象急促,说明表症未解。如果出现气喘、出汗等症,宜用葛根黄芩黄连汤主治。

Differentiation of pulse and syndrome / pattern [related to] taiyang disease and treatment (part 2)

【英译】

Line 34

[The syndrome/pattern of] taiyang disease [pertains to] the one [to be treated by] Gegen Guizhi [Decoction] (葛根桂枝汤, pueraria and cinnamon twig decoction). [When] wrongly treated by purgation，[it will cause] constant diarrhea and rapid pulse，[indicating that] the external [syndrome/pattern is] not relieved. [If there are symptoms and signs of] panting and sweating，Gegen Huangqin Huanglian Decoction (葛根黄芩黄连汤，pueraria, scutellaria and coptis decoction) [can be used to] treat it.

Gegen Huangqin Huanglian Decoction (葛根黄芩黄连汤，pueraria，scutellaria and coptis decoction) [is composed of] 0.5 *jin* of Gegen (葛根，pueraria，Radix Puerariae)，2 *liang* of Gancao (甘草，licorice，Radix Glycyrrhizae Praeparata) (broiled)，2 *liang* of Huangqin (黄芩，scutellaria，Radix Scutellariae) and 3 *liang* of Huanglian (黄连，coptis，Rhizoma Coptidis).

These four ingredients [can be decocted in] 8 *sheng* of water. Gegen (葛根，pueraria，Radix Puerariae) is decocted first to reduce 2 *sheng* [of water]. [Then] the rest medicinals are put into [it to decoct and to get] 2 *sheng* [after] boiling. The dregs are removed and [the decoction is] taken warm for twice.

【原文】

(三五)

太阳病,头痛,发热,身疼,腰痛,骨节疼痛,恶风,无汗而喘者,麻黄汤主之。

麻黄汤方

麻黄三两(去节)、桂枝二两(去皮)、甘草一两(炙)、杏仁七十个(去皮尖)。

右四味,以水九升,先煮麻黄,减二升,去上沫,内诸药,煮取二升半,去滓,温服八合,覆取微似汗,不须啜粥,余如桂枝法将息。

【今译】

太阳病,患者头痛、发热、身体疼痛,腰痛,关节疼痛,恶风,无汗而气喘,脉浮紧,宜用麻黄汤主治。

【原文】

(三六)

太阳与阳明合病,喘而胸满者,不可下,宜麻黄汤。

【今译】

太阳与阳明合病,患者气喘,胸部胀闷,不可用攻下法,宜用麻黄汤主治。

Differentiation of pulse and syndrome/pattern [related to] taiyang disease and treatment (part 2)

【英译】

Line 35

Taiyang disease, [characterized by] headache, fever, body pain, lumbago, arthralgia, aversion to wind, no sweating and panting, [can be] treated by Mahuang Decoction (麻黄汤, dephedra decoction).

Mahuang Decoction (麻黄汤, dephedra decoction) [is composed of] 3 *liang* of Mahuang (麻黄, ephedra, Herba Ephedrae) (nodes-removed), 2 *liang* of Guizhi (桂枝, cinnamon twig, Ramulus Cinnamomi) (bark-removed), 1 *liang* of Gancao (甘草, licorice, Radix Glycyrrhizae Praeparata) (broiled) and 70 pieces of Xingren (杏仁, apricot kernel, Semen Armeniacae Amarum) (peel-and-tips-removed).

The four ingredients mentioned above [are decocted] in 9 *sheng* of water. Mahuang (麻黄, ephedra, Herba Ephedrae) is decocted first to reduce 2 *sheng* [of water]. The foam is removed and other ingredients are put into [it to decoct and to get] 2.5 *sheng* [of water after] boiling. The dregs are removed and [the decoction is] taken warm 8 *ge* [each time]. [Then the patient is] covered [with quilt or clothes to] induce light sweating without any need to take porridge. Contraindications are the same as that for Guizhi [Decoction] (桂枝汤, cinnamon twig decoction).

【英译】

Line 36

Disease [due to invasion of pathogenic factors into] both taiyang [meridian] and yangming [meridian] causes panting and chest fullness, [which] should be treated by Mahuang Decoction (麻黄汤, dephedra decoction), not by purgation.

【原文】

(三七)

太阳病,十日以去,脉浮细而嗜卧者,外已解也,设胸满胁痛者,与小柴胡汤;脉但浮者,与麻黄汤。

小柴胡汤方

柴胡半斤,黄芩、人参、甘草(炙)、生姜各三两(切),大枣十二枚,半夏半斤(洗)。

右七味,以水一斗二升,煮取六升,取滓,再煮取三升,温服一升,日三服。

【今译】

太阳病,十日之后,患者脉浮细,嗜卧,说明外感症候已解,如果胸满胁痛,可用小柴胡汤治疗。但如果脉浮,则可用麻黄汤主治。

*Differentiation of pulse and syndrome/pattern
[related to] taiyang disease and treatment (part 2)*

【英译】

Line 37

Taiyang disease, after ten days [of treatment and marked by] floating and thin pulse and somnolence, [indicates that] the external [syndrome/pattern is] already relieved. [If there are symptoms and signs of] chest fullness and costal pain, [it can be treated] by Xiao Chaihu Decoction (小柴胡汤, minor bupleurum decoction). [If] the pulse is floating, Mahuang Decoction (麻黄汤, dephedra decoction) [can be] used.

Xiao Chaihu Decoction (小柴胡汤, minor bupleurum decoction) [is composed of] 0.5 *jin* of Chaihu (柴胡, bupleurum, Radix Bupleuri), 3 *liang* of Huangqin (黄芩, scutellaria, Radix Scutellariae), 3 *liang* of Renshen (人参, ginseng, Radix Ginseng), 3 *liang* of Gancao (甘草, licorice, Radix Glycyrrhizae Praeparata) (broiled), 3 *liang* of Shengjiang (生姜, fresh ginger, Rhizoma Zingiberis Recens) (cut), 12 pieces of Dazao (大枣, jujube, Fructus Ziziphus Jujubae) and 0.5 *sheng* of Banxia (半夏, pinellia, Rhizoma Pinelliae) (washed).

The seven ingredients mentioned above [are decocted] in 1.2 *dou* of water and get 6 *sheng* [after] boiling. [After] removal of the dregs, [the decoction is] boiled again to get 3 *sheng* [of water]. [The decoction is] taken warm 1 *sheng* [each time] and three times a day.

【原文】

(三八)

太阳中风,脉浮紧,发热,恶寒,身疼痛,不汗出而烦躁者,大青龙汤主之。若脉微弱,汗出恶风者,不可服之,服之则厥逆,筋惕肉瞤,此为逆也。

大青龙汤方

麻黄六两(去节)、桂枝二两(去皮)、甘草二两(炙)、杏仁四十枚(去皮尖)、生姜三两(切)、大枣十二枚(擘)、石膏如鸡子大(碎)。

右七味,以水九升,先煮麻黄,减二升,去上沫,纳诸药,煮取三升,去滓,温服一升,取微似汗,汗出多者,温粉粉之。一服汗者,停后服,汗多亡阳,遂虚,恶风烦躁,不得眠也。

【今译】

太阳中风证,有脉象浮紧、发热、恶寒、全身疼痛、汗不得出、烦躁不安等症状,可用大青龙汤主治疗。如果有脉象微弱、汗出恶风等症状,不可用大青龙汤治疗。若误用了,就会引发四肢厥冷、筋肉颤动,这是误治而造成的后果。

Differentiation of pulse and syndrome / pattern [related to] taiyang disease and treatment (part 2)

【英译】

Line 38

Taiyang [disease with] wind attack, [characterized by] floating and tight pulse, fever, aversion to cold, body pain, no sweating and dysphoria, [can be] treated by Da Qinglong Decoction (大青龙汤, major blue loong decoction). If [there are symptoms and signs of] light and weak pulse, sweating and aversion to wind, [this decoction] cannot be used. [If] used, [it will cause] reversal cold [of the limbs] and spasm of sinews and muscles. This is [the result of] mistreatment.

Da Qinglong Decoction (大青龙汤, major blue loong decoction) [is composed of] 6 *liang* of Mahuang (麻黄, ephedra, Herba Ephedrae) (nodes-removed), 2 *liang* of Guizhi (桂枝, cinnamon twig, Ramulus Cinnamomi) (bark-removed), 2 *liang* of Gancao (甘草, licorice, Radix Glycyrrhizae Praeparata) (broiled), 40 pieces of Xingren (杏仁, apricot kernel, Semen Armeniacae Amarum) (peel-and-tips-removed), 3 *liang* of Shengjiang (生姜, fresh ginger, Rhizoma Zingiberis Recens) (cut), 10 pieces of Dazao (大枣, jujube, Fructus Ziziphus Jujubae) (broken) and Shigao (石膏, gypsum, Gypsum Fibrosum) (as big as an egg and to be broken for decoction).

These seven ingredients mentioned above [are decocted] in 9 *sheng* of water. Mahuang (麻黄, ephedra, Herba Ephedrae) is decocted first to reduce 2 *sheng* [of water]. The foam is removed and other ingredients are put into [it to decoct and get] 3 *sheng* [after] boiling. The dregs are removed and [the decoction is] taken warm 1 *sheng* [each time] to induce light sweating. [If] sweating is profuse, blend warm rice powder [can be used to] relieve sweating. [If] sweating [is induced after] the first time of taking [the decoction], [it] cannot be taken again. Otherwise [it will cause] profuse sweating and loss of yang, [consequently leading to] deficiency, aversion to wind, dysphoria and insomnia.

【原文】

(三九)

伤寒脉浮缓,身不疼,但重,乍有轻时,无少阴证者,大青龙汤发之。

【今译】

伤寒病,患者脉象浮缓,身体不痛,但很沉重,偶尔有所减轻,没有少阴证的表现,可用大青龙汤发汗解表。

【原文】

(四〇)

伤寒表不解,心下有水气,干呕,发热而咳,或渴,或利,或噎,或小便不利,少腹满,或喘者,小青龙汤主之。

小青龙汤方

麻黄(去节)、芍药、细辛、干姜、甘草(炙)、桂枝各三两(去皮),五味子半升,半夏半升(洗)。

右八味,以水一斗,先煮麻黄,减二升,去上沫,内诸药,煮取三升,去滓,温服一升。若渴,去半夏加栝楼根三两。若微利,去麻黄加荛花如一鸡子熬令赤色。若噎者,去麻黄加附子一枚炮。若小便不利少腹

Differentiation of pulse and syndrome / pattern [related to] taiyang disease and treatment (part 2)

【英译】

Line 39

[Disease caused by] cold damage，[characterized by] floating and slow pulse without pain of the body and shaoyin syndrome/pattern but [with] heaviness [of the body]，[can be] treated by Da Qinglong Decoction（大青龙汤，major blue loong decoction）.

【英译】

Line 40

[Disease caused by] cold damage，[characterized by] no relief of external [syndrome/pattern]，retention of water，retching，fever with cough，or thirst，or diarrhea，or hiccup，or dysuria，lower abdominal fullness，or panting，[can be] treated by Xiao Qinglong Decoction（小青龙汤，minor blue loong decoction）.

Xiao Qinglong Decoction（小青龙汤，minor blue loong decoction）[is composed of] 3 *liang* of Mahuang（麻黄，ephedra，Herba Ephedrae）（nodes-removed），3 *liang* of Shaoyao（芍药，peony，Radix Paeoniae），3 *liang* of Xixin（细辛，asarum，Herba Asari），3 *liang* of Ganjiang（干姜，dried ginger，Rhizoma Zingiberis），3 *liang* of Gancao（甘草，licorice，Radix Glycyrrhizae Praeparata）（broiled）and 3 *liang* of Guizhi（桂枝，cinnamon twig，Ramulus Cinnamomi）（bark-removed），0.5 *sheng* of Wuweizi（五味子，Chinese magnoliavine，Fructus Schisandrae Chinensis）and 0.5 *sheng* of Banxia（半夏，pinellia，Rhizoma Pinelliae）（washed）.

These eight ingredients mentioned above [are decocted] in 1 *dou* of water. Mahuang（麻黄，ephedra，Herba Ephedrae）is

满者,去麻黄加茯苓四两。若喘,去麻黄加杏仁半升去皮尖。且荛花不治利,麻黄主喘,今此语反之,疑非仲景意。

【今译】

伤寒病,其表症未解,心胸之下有水饮,患者有发热、或干呕、或咳嗽,或口渴,或小便不利,或少腹满,或气喘等症状,可用小青龙汤治疗。

【原文】

(四一)

伤寒,心下有水气,咳而微喘,发热不渴,服汤已,渴者,此寒去欲解也,小青龙汤主之。

【今译】

伤寒病,心下有水饮停聚,患者有咳嗽、微喘、发热、不渴等症状。如果服用汤药后出现口渴,说明外寒祛除,内饮得解。可用小青龙汤治疗。

Differentiation of pulse and syndrome/pattern [related to] taiyang disease and treatment (part 2)

decocted first to reduce 2 *sheng* [of water]. The foam is removed and other ingredients are put into [it to decoct and to get] 3 *sheng* [after] boiling. The dregs are removed and [the decoction is] taken warm 1 *sheng* [each time]. If [there is] thirst, Banxia (半夏, pinellia, Rhizoma Pinelliae) is removed and 3 *liang* of Gualougen (栝楼根, trichosanthes root, Radix Trichosanthis) is added; if [there is] slight diarrhea, Mahuang (麻黄, ephedra, Herba Ephedrae) is removed and Raohua (荛花, canescent wikstroemia, Wikstroemia Canescens) is added (as big as an egg and is stewed till turning red); if [there is] hiccup, Mahuang (麻黄, ephedra, Herba Ephedrae) is removed and 1 piece of processed Fuzi (附子, aconite, Radix Aconiti Lateralis Preparata) (fried heavily) is added; if [there are] dysuria and lower abdominal fullness, Mahuang (麻黄, ephedra, Herba Ephedrae) is removed and 4 *liang* of Fuling (茯苓, poria, Poria) is added; if [there is] panting, Mahuang (麻黄, ephedra, Herba Ephedrae) is removed and 0.5 *sheng* of Xingren (杏仁, apricot kernel, Semen Armeniacae Amarum) (peel-and-tips-removed) is added.

【英译】

Line 41

Cold damage, [characterized by] retention of water in the epigastrium, cough, slight panting, fever and hydroadipsia, [can be] treated by [Xiao Qinglong] Decoction (小青龙汤, minor blue loong decoction). [If there is] thirst [after taking the decoction], it [indicates that] cold is relieved and [the disease is] about to heal.

【原文】

(四二)

太阳病,外证未解,脉浮弱者,当以汗解,宜桂枝汤。

【今译】

太阳病,表证未解,脉象浮弱,仍可用汗法治疗,宜用桂枝汤主治。

【原文】

(四三)

太阳病,下之微喘者,表未解故也,桂枝加厚朴杏子汤主之。

【今译】

太阳病,如用攻下法治疗,则会引起轻度气喘,表证没有解除,可用桂枝加厚朴杏仁汤治疗。

【原文】

(四四)

太阳病,外证未解,不可下也,下之为逆。欲解外者,宜桂枝汤。

【今译】

太阳病,表证没有解除时,不可用泻下法。如果使用了泻下法,就属误治。宜用桂枝汤主治。

Differentiation of pulse and syndrome/pattern [related to] taiyang disease and treatment（part 2）

【英译】

Line 42

Taiyang disease，[characterized by] failure to relieve external syndrome/pattern，floating and weak pulse，should [be treated] by diaphoresis with Guizhi Decoction （桂枝汤，cinnamon twig decoction）.

【英译】

Line 43

Taiyang disease，[characterized by] light panting and failure to relieve external [syndrome/pattern due to mistreatment with] purgation，[can be] treated by Guizhi Decoction （桂枝汤，cinnamon twig decoction）with addition of Houpo (厚朴，magnolia bark，Cortex Magnoliae Officinalis）and Xingzi（杏子，apricot kernel，Semen Armeniacae Amarum）.

【英译】

Line 44

Taiyang disease without relieving external syndrome/pattern cannot [be treated by] purgation. [To use] purgation is a mistreatment. To relieve external [syndrome/pattern]，Guizhi Decoction (桂枝汤，cinnamon twig decoction）should [be used].

【原文】

(四五)

太阳病,先发汗不解,而复下之,脉浮者不愈。浮为在外,而反下之,故令不愈。今脉浮,故在外,当须解外则愈,宜桂枝汤。

【今译】

太阳病,先用发汗法,但外感症候未解。因而又用攻下的方法,脉象仍浮,则病未治愈。脉象浮说明病邪在表,这就是泻下法不能治愈的缘故。如今脉象浮,所以病邪在表,只有解表才能治愈疾病,宜用桂枝汤主治。

【原文】

(四六)

太阳病,脉浮紧,无汗,发热,身疼痛,八九日不解,表证仍在,此当发其汗。服药已微除,其人发烦目瞑,剧者必衄。衄乃解,所以然者,阳气重故也,麻黄汤主之。

【今译】

太阳病,脉象浮紧,无汗,发热,全身疼痛,八九天后依然不解,表证仍存在,这种情况下应通过发汗治疗。服用汤药后病症略有缓解,患者烦躁、目眩,病情严重的必然出现鼻衄。鼻衄出现后病情必然有所缓解,之所以如此,是因为阳气重的缘故,宜用麻黄汤主治。

Differentiation of pulse and syndrome／pattern ［related to］ taiyang disease and treatment（part 2）

【英译】

Line 45

［External syndrome/pattern in］ taiyang disease is not relieved ［after application of］ diaphoresis first. ［If treated by］ purgation again，［it will］ not heal ［if］ the pulse is floating. Floating ［pulse indicates that the disease is］ in the external，［that is why］ purgation cannot heal ［it］. Though ［wrongly treated by purgation，］ the pulse ［is still］ floating because ［the disease is located］ in the external and should ［be treated by］ Guizhi Decoction（桂枝汤，cinnamon twig decoction）to relieve the external and heal ［the disease］.

【英译】

Line 46

Taiyang disease，［characterized by］ floating and tight pulse，no sweating，fever，body pain，failure to relieve after eight or nine days of procrastination and existence of external syndrome/pattern，it should ［be treated by］ diaphoresis. ［The disease will be］ slightly alleviated after taking ［Mahuang Decoction（麻黄汤，Ephedra Decoction）］. ［But］ the patient ［still feels］ dysphoric and tired to open the eyes. ［If］ severe，［it will cause］ epistaxis. ［Only when there is］ epistaxis ［can the disease be］ relieved ［for］ yang qi is restored.

【原文】

(四七)

太阳病,脉浮紧,发热,身无汗,自衄者愈。

【今译】

太阳病,脉象浮紧,身体发热,全身无汗,有鼻衄出现的,则会痊愈。

【原文】

(四八)

二阳并病,太阳初得病时,发其汗,汗先出不彻,因转属阳明,续自微汗出,不恶寒。若太阳病证不罢者,不可下,下之为逆,如此可小发汗。设面色缘缘正赤者,阳气怫郁在表,当解之、熏之。若发汗不彻,不足言,阳气怫郁不得越,当汗不汗,其人躁烦,不知痛处,乍在腹中,乍在四肢,按之不可得,其人短气但坐,以汗出不彻故也,更发汗则愈。何以知汗出不彻? 以脉涩故知也。

【今译】

太阳与阳明并病,太阳经初发病时,可通过发汗法治疗,但汗先发的并不透彻,因而转入阳明经,续而微汗自出,无恶寒之状。如果太阳病证没有缓解,不可使用下法,使用下法之为误治,这时可小发汗。如果患者面色彤彤发红,阳气瘀滞在表,应当通过发汗予以解除,通过熏蒸予以治疗。如果发汗不透彻,无成效,阳气郁滞而不得外越,应当出汗但却没有出汗,患者躁烦,痛处不明,或在腹中,或在四肢,无法通过按压确定,患者气短,只想坐着,都是因为汗出不透彻的缘故,只有继续发汗才能痊愈。如何知道汗出不透彻呢? 脉涩就是明证。

Differentiation of pulse and syndrome/pattern [related to] taiyang disease and treatment (part 2)

【英译】

Line 47

Taiyang disease, [characterized by] floating and tight pulse, fever and no sweating, will heal [if] epistaxis [occurs] spontaneously.

【英译】

Line 48

Disease involving both taiyang [meridian] and yangming [meridian is caused by treatment for] diaphoresis at the early stage without [inducing] thorough sweating, [which eventually] transmits into yangming [meridian] and consequently leads to slight sweating without aversion to cold. If the syndrome/pattern of taiyang disease is not alleviated, purgation cannot be used, [because] it is a mistreatment, [the problem caused by which can be] solved by [treatment] for slight perspiration. [If the patient's] face turns red, [it is caused by] stagnation of pathogenic factors in the superficies [which can be] relieved by diaphoresis and fumigation. If perspiration is not thorough, [there appear symptoms and signs like] unclear tenderness, stagnation of pathogenic factors in the superficies, failure to induce sweating, dysphoria, unclear location of pain [which is] either in the abdomen or in the four limbs, and inability to clarify through palpation. The patient feels difficult to breathe and wants to sit due to thorough perspiration. If perspiration is promoted, [the disease will be] healed. How to know whether perspiration is thorough or not? Uneven pulse is the possible way to understand.

【原文】

（四九）

脉浮数者，法当汗出而愈。若下之，身重心悸者，不可发汗，当自汗出乃解。所以然者，尺中脉微，此里虚。须表里实，津液自和，便自汗出愈。

【今译】

脉象浮数的，应当通过发汗祛除邪气而治愈。如果误用了下法，导致身体沉重和心悸，就不可再用汗法。只有自行汗出病情才能得到解除。之所以这样，是因为尺脉微弱，这是里气不足的表现。只有表里之气恢复，津液自和，才会自动出汗，从而使疾病得以痊愈。

【原文】

（五〇）

脉浮紧者，法当身疼痛，宜以汗解之。假令尺中迟者，不可发汗。何以知之然？以营气不足，血少故也。

【今译】

脉象浮紧，身体应有出现疼痛之症，宜用发汗法解表。如果尺脉迟，则不能用汗法。为什么呢？因为营气不足、阴血虚少。

Differentiation of pulse and syndrome/pattern
[related to] taiyang disease and treatment (part 2)

【英译】

Line 49

[If] the pulse is floating and rapid, [it can be] improved by diaphoresis. If purgation is used, [it will cause] heaviness of the body and palpitation [which] cannot [be treated by] diaphoresis. Only spontaneous sweating can relieve [it]. That is why slight [beating of] the pulse in the chi [pulse] shows weakness. [If there is] excessive [pathogenic factors in] the internal and external, [if] fluid and humor are in harmony, spontaneous sweating [will naturally] heal [the disease].

【英译】

Line 50

Floating and tight pulse certainly indicates pain of the body and can be relieved by diaphoresis. If the pulse in the chi [pulse] is slow, sweating cannot be induced. What is the reason? Because nutrient qi is insufficient and blood is not enough.

【原文】

(五一)

脉浮者,病在表,可发汗,宜麻黄汤。

【今译】

脉象浮的,说明病邪在表,可通过发汗治疗。宜用麻黄汤主治。

【原文】

(五二)

脉浮而数者,可发汗,宜麻黄汤。

【今译】

脉象浮而数的,可通过发汗治疗,宜用麻黄汤主治。

【原文】

(五三)

病常自汗出者,此为营气和,营气和者,外不谐,以卫气不共营气谐和故尔。以营行脉中,卫行脉外,复发其汗,荣卫和则愈,宜桂枝汤。

【今译】

患者常自汗出的,是营气和的表现。但营气虽和,卫气却不和谐,正是由于卫气不能与营气谐和,因此患者常自汗出。由于营气行于脉中,卫气行于脉外,可以再用发汗法,从而使营卫趋于谐和,使疾病得以痊愈,宜用桂枝汤主治。

Differentiation of pulse and syndrome/pattern
[related to] taiyang disease and treatment（part 2）

【英译】

Line 51

Floating pulse [indicates that] the disease is in the external and can be treated by diaphoresis with Mahuang Decoction（麻黄汤，Ephedra Decoction）.

【英译】

Line 52

[The disease] with floating and rapid pulse can [be treated by] diaphoresis with Mahuang Decoction（麻黄汤，Ephedra Decoction）.

【英译】

Line 53

Disease with spontaneous sweating indicates [failure of] nutrient qi [to control the internal] and [defense qi] to protect the external，consequently causing disharmony due to imbalance between defense qi and nutrient qi. Since nutrient qi flows in the vessels and defense qi flows outside the vessels，perspiration will harmonize the functions of both with Guizhi Decoction（桂枝汤，cinnamon twig decoction）.

【原文】

(五四)

病人脏无他病,时发热、自汗出而不愈者,此卫气不和也。先其时发汗则愈,宜桂枝汤。

【今译】

病人内脏没有其他疾病,时而发热,自汗出而不能痊愈的,是由于卫气不和的缘故。可在病人发热出汗之前用发汗法治疗,病就可愈。宜用桂枝汤主治。

【原文】

(五五)

伤寒脉浮紧,不发汗,因致衄者,麻黄汤主之。

【今译】

伤寒病,脉象浮紧,但没有发汗,因而造成鼻衄,可用麻黄汤治疗。

Differentiation of pulse and syndrome/pattern [related to] taiyang disease and treatment (part 2)

【英译】

Line 54

The patient has no problems in the viscera，[but there are] fever and spontaneous sweating. [It is] unable to heal. This [is caused by] disharmony of defense qi [and can be] healed by diaphoresis with Guizhi Decoction （桂枝汤，cinnamon twig decoction）before the patient has a fever and sweating.

【英译】

Line 55

[The disease caused by] cold damage with floating and tight pulse and without perspiration causes epistaxis and can be treated by Mahuang Decoction（麻黄汤，Ephedra Decoction）.

【原文】

（五六）

伤寒不大便六七日，头痛有热者，与承气汤。其小便清者，知不在里，仍在表也，当须发汗。若头痛者，必衄，宜桂枝汤。

【今译】

伤寒病，患者六七日不大便，头痛，发热，可用承气汤治疗。其小便清长的，说明邪不在里，仍在其表，应当通过发汗治疗。如果头痛，则必然引发鼻衄，宜用桂枝汤主治。

【原文】

（五七）

伤寒发汗已解，半日许复烦，脉浮数者，可更发汗，宜桂枝汤。

【今译】

伤寒病，发汗后表证已解，大约过了半天病人又开始感到烦躁，脉象浮数，可以再行发汗，宜用桂枝汤主治。

Differentiation of pulse and syndrome / pattern [related to] taiyang disease and treatment（part 2）

【英译】

Line 56

[The disease caused by] cold damage，[characterized by] difficulty in defecation in six to seven days，headache and fever，[can be treated] by Chengqi Decoction（承气汤，decoction for harmonizing qi）. [If] urine is clear，[it indicates that pathogenic heat] is not in the internal but in the external, and [can be treated by] diaphoresis. If there is headache，[it will] cause epistaxis and can [be treated by] Guizhi Decoction（桂枝汤，cinnamon twig decoction）.

【英译】

Line 57

[The disease caused by] cold damage with perspiration already relieved，[characterized by] dysphoria [occurring] half a day later，floating and rapid pulse，can [be treated by] diaphoresis with Guizhi Decoction（桂枝汤，cinnamon twig decoction）.

【原文】

(五八)

凡病,若发汗,若吐,若下,若亡血,亡津液,阴阳自和者,必自愈。

【今译】

任何疾病,如果用发汗法治疗,或用涌吐法治疗,或用泻下法治疗,若导致血液耗伤、津液伤亡的,如果阴阳能自相调和,疾病就一定能痊愈。

【原文】

(五九)

大下之后,复发汗,小便不利者,亡津液故也。勿治之,得少便利,必自愈。

【今译】

通过峻烈的泻下之后,如果又用发汗法,导致小便不利的,是因为津液受了损伤。不可用利小便之法治疗,津液恢复后小便自利的,就可自愈了。

【原文】

(六〇)

下之后,复发汗,必振寒,脉微细。所以然者,以内外俱虚故也。

【今译】

使用泻下法之后,又用发汗法,必然引发畏寒战栗,脉象微细。之所以引起这样的变化,是内外俱虚的缘故。

*Differentiation of pulse and syndrome / pattern
[related to] taiyang disease and treatment (part 2)*

【英译】

Line 58

Any disease, [characterized by] sweating, or vomiting, or diarrhea, or hemorrhage, or loss of fluid and humor, will heal spontaneously [when] yin and yang are harmonized naturally.

【英译】

Line 59

Perspiration [occurring] again after [application of] purgation with dysuria is caused by loss of fluid and humor. [Such a case] should not be treated [by promoting urination]. [It] will heal spontaneously [when] urination is normalized.

【英译】

Line 60

Perspiration [occurs] again after [application of] purgation [with] aversion to cold, chilliness, light and thin pulse, the cause [of which is wrong application of purgation that results in] dual deficiency of the internal and external.

【原文】

(六一)

下之后,复发汗,昼日烦躁不得眠,夜而安静,不呕、不渴、无表证,脉沉微,身无大热者,干姜附子汤主之。

干姜附子汤方

干姜一两、附子一枚(生用,去皮,破八片)。

右二味,以水三升,煮取一升,去滓顿服。

【今译】

使用泻下法之后,又用发汗法,致使病人白天烦躁,不能安睡,但夜晚安静;不作呕,不口渴,无表症,脉象沉微,身上没有大热的,宜用干姜附子汤治疗。

Differentiation of pulse and syndrome / pattern [related to] taiyang disease and treatment (part 2)

【英译】

Line 61

Perspiration, [occurring] again after [application of] purgation, [characterized by] insomnia due to dysphoria in the daytime, quietness at night, no nausea, no thirst, no external syndrome/pattern, light and deep pulse, and no severe fever, [can be] treated by Ganjiang Fuzi Decoction (干姜附子汤, dried ginger and radix aconiti carmichaeli decoction).

Ganjiang Fuzi Decoction (干姜附子汤, dried ginger and radix aconiti carmichaeli decoction) [is composed of] 1 *liang* of Ganjiang (干姜, dried ginger, Rhizoma Zingiberis) and 1 piece of Fuzi (附子, aconite, Radix Aconiti Lateralis Preparata) (fresh, remove the bark and break into eight small pieces).

These two ingredients are decocted in 3 *sheng* of water to get 1 *sheng* [after boiling]. [After] removal of the dregs, [the decoction is] taken warm.

【原文】

(六二)

发汗后，身疼痛，脉沉迟者，桂枝加芍药生姜各一两，人参三两新加汤主之。

桂枝加芍药生姜人参新加汤方

桂枝三两(去皮)、芍药四两、甘草二两(炙)、人参三两、大枣十二枚(擘)、生姜四两。

右六味，以水一斗二升煮取三升，去滓，温服一升。本云桂枝汤，今加芍药生姜人参。

【今译】

使用发汗法之后，患者身体疼痛，脉象沉迟，宜用桂枝加芍药生姜各一两，人参三两新加汤主治。

Differentiation of pulse and syndrome / pattern [related to] taiyang disease and treatment (part 2)

【英译】

Line 62

[The disease, characterized by] generalized pain and deep and slow pulse after diaphoresis, [can be] treated by Guizhi Decoction (桂枝汤, cinnamon twig decoction) added with Shaoyao (芍药, peony, Radix Paeoniae), Shengjiang (生姜, fresh ginger, Rhizoma Zingiberis Recens) and Renshen (人参, ginseng, Radix Ginseng).

Guizhi Decoction (桂枝汤, cinnamon twig decoction) added with Shaoyao (芍药, peony, Radix Paeoniae), Shengjiang (生姜, fresh ginger, Rhizoma Zingiberis Recens) and Renshen (人参, ginseng, Radix Ginseng) [is composed of] 3 *liang* of Guizhi (桂枝, cinnamon twig, Ramulus Cinnamomi) (bark-removed), 4 *liang* of Shaoyao (芍药, peony, Radix Paeoniae), 2 *liang* of Gancao (甘草, licorice, Radix Glycirrhizae Praeparata) (broiled), 3 *liang* of Renshen (人参, ginseng, Radix Ginseng), 12 pieces of Dazao (大枣, jujube, Fructus Ziziphus Jujubae) (broken) and 4 *liang* of Shengjiang (生姜, fresh ginger, Rhizoma Zingiberis Recens).

These six ingredients are decocted in 1 *dou* and 2 *sheng* of water to get 3 *sheng* [after] boiling. The dregs are removed and [the decoction is] taken warm 1 *sheng* [each time]. The old edition says that Guizhi Decoction (桂枝汤, cinnamon twig decoction) is added with Shaoyao (芍药, peony, Radix Paeoniae), Shengjiang (生姜, fresh ginger, Rhizoma Zingiberis Recens) and Renshen (人参, ginseng, Radix Ginseng).

【原文】

(六三)

发汗后,不可更行桂枝汤,汗出而喘,无大热者,可与麻黄杏仁甘草石膏汤。

麻黄杏仁甘草石膏汤方

麻黄四两(去节)、杏仁五十个(去皮尖)、甘草二两(炙)、石膏半斤(碎,绵裹)。

右四味,以水七升,煮麻黄减二升,去上沫,内诸药,煮取二升,去滓,温服一升,本云黄耳杯。

【今译】

发汗以后,不能再用桂枝汤,出现汗出,气喘,无大热症状的,宜用麻黄杏仁甘草石膏汤治疗。

Differentiation of pulse and syndrome / pattern
[related to] taiyang disease and treatment (part 2)

【英译】

Line 63

[The disease] after perspiration cannot be treated by Guizhi Decoction (桂枝汤, cinnamon twig decoction). [If there are symptoms and signs of] sweating, panting and light fever, [it] can be treated by Mahuang Xingren Gancao Shigao Decoction (麻黄杏仁甘草石膏汤, ephedra, apricot kernel, licorice and gypsum decoction).

Mahuang Xingren Gancao Shigao Decoction (麻黄杏仁甘草石膏汤, ephedra, apricot kernel, licorice and gypsum decoction) [is composed of] 4 *liang* of Mahuang (麻黄, ephedra, Herba Ephedrae) (nodes-removed), 50 pieces of Xingren (杏仁, apricot kernel, Semen Armeniacae Amarum) (peel-and-tips-removed), 2 *liang* of Gancao (甘草, licorice, Radix Glycyrrhizae Praeparata) (broiled) and 0.5 *jin* of Shigao (石膏, gypsum, Gypsum Fibrosum) (to be broken into small pieces and wrapped in a cotton gauze).

These four ingredients mentioned above [can be decocted] in 7 *sheng* of water. Mahuang (麻黄, ephedra, Herba Ephedrae) is decocted [first] to reduce 2 *sheng* [of water]. [After] removal of the foam, other ingredients are put into [it] and decocted to get 2 *sheng* [after] boiling. The dregs are removed and [the decoction is] taken warm 1 *sheng* [each time].

【原文】

(六四)

发汗过多,其人叉手自冒心,心下悸,欲得按者,桂枝甘草汤主之。

桂枝甘草汤方

桂枝四两(去皮)、甘草二两(炙)。

右二味,以水三升,煮取一升,去滓,顿服。

【今译】

发汗太多,令患者双手交叉按着心胸,心悸不安,只有用手按压方感舒适,宜用桂枝甘草汤治疗。

【原文】

(六五)

发汗后,其人脐下悸者,欲作奔豚,茯苓桂枝甘草大枣汤主之。

茯苓桂枝甘草大枣汤方

茯苓半斤,桂枝四两(去皮)、甘草二两(炙)、大枣十五枚(擘)。

右四味,以甘澜水一斗,先煮茯苓,减二升,内诸药,煮取三升,去

Differentiation of pulse and syndrome / pattern [related to] taiyang disease and treatment (part 2)

【英译】

Line 64

[Due to] profuse sweating, the patient presses the chest with folded hands [in order to alleviate] palpitation, [which can be] treated by Guizhi Gancao Deccotion (桂枝甘草汤, cinnamon twig and licorice decoction).

Guizhi Gancao Deccotion (桂枝甘草汤, cinnamon twig and dry licorice decoction) [is composed of] 4 *liang* of Guizhi (桂枝, cinnamon twig, Ramulus Cinnamomi) (bark-removed) and 2 *liang* of Gancao (甘草, licorice, Radix Glycyrrhizae Praeparata) (broiled).

These two ingredients are decocted in 3 *sheng* of water to get 1 *sheng* [after] boiling. The dregs are removed and [the decoction is] taken once the whole.

【英译】

Line 65

After diaphoresis, the patient suffers from palpitation underneath the navel similar to a running piglet [which can be] treated by Fuling Guizhi Gancao Dazao Decoction (茯苓桂枝甘草大枣汤, poria, cinnamon twig, licorice and jujube decoction).

Fuling Guizhi Gancao Dazao Decoction (茯苓桂枝甘草大枣汤, poria, cinnamon twig, licorice and jujube decoction) [is composed of] 0.5 *jin* of Fuling (茯苓, poria, Poria), 4 *liang* of Guizhi (桂枝, cinnamon twig, Ramulus Cinnamomi) (bark-removed), 2 *liang* of Gancao (甘草, licorice, Radix Glycyrrhizae Praeparata) (broiled) and 15 pieces of Dazao (大枣, jujube, Fructus Ziziphus Jujubae) (broken).

These four ingredients are decocted in 1 *dou* of Ganlan water

滓,温服一升,日三服。作甘澜水法:取水二升,置大盆内,以杓扬之,水上有珠子五六千颗相逐,取用之。

【今译】

使用发汗法以后,患者出现脐下颤动不宁,如奔豚欲将发作,宜用茯苓桂枝甘草大枣汤治疗。

【原文】

(六六)

发汗后,腹胀满者,厚朴生姜半夏甘草人参汤主之。

厚朴生姜半夏甘草人参汤方

厚朴半斤(炙,去皮)、生姜半斤(切)、半夏半升(洗)、甘草二两、人参一两。

右五味,以水一斗,煮取三升,去滓,温服一升,日三服。

Differentiation of pulse and syndrome / pattern [related to] taiyang disease and treatment (part 2)

(repeatedly pumped up water). Fuling (茯苓, poria, *Poria*) is decocted first to reduce 2 *sheng* [of water]. [Then] other ingredients are put into it to decoct to get 3 *sheng* [after] boiling. The dregs are removed and [the decoction is] taken warm 1 *sheng* [each time] and 3 times a day. To produce Ganlan water, 2 *dou* of water is put into a large basin and repeatedly pumped up with a spoon. [When there are] over five to six thousands of bubbles [popping up] over the surface of water, [it becomes Ganlan water and] can be used [to decoct these ingredients].

【英译】

Line 66

After diaphoresis, abdominal distension and fullness [can be] treated by Houpo Shengjiang Banxia Gancao Renshen Decoction (厚朴生姜半夏甘草人参汤, magnolica bark, fresh ginger, pinellia, licorice and ginseng decoction).

Houpo Shengjiang Banxia Gancao Renshen Decoction (厚朴生姜半夏甘草人参汤, magnolica bark, fresh ginger, pinellia, licorice and ginseng decoction) [is composed of] 0.5 *jin* of Houpo (厚朴, magnolia bark, Cortex Magnoliae Officinalis) (broiled, peel-removed), 0.5 *jin* of Shengjiang (生姜, fresh ginger, Rhizoma Zingiberis Recens) (cut), 0.5 *jin* of Banxia (半夏, pinellia, Rhizoma Pinelliae) (washed), 2 *liang* of Gancao (甘草, licorice, Radix Glycyrrhizae Praeparata) and 1 *liang* of Renshen (人参, ginseng, Radix Ginseng).

These five ingredients are deocted in 1 *dou* of water to get 3 *sheng* [after] boiling. The dregs are removed and [the decoction is] taken warm 1 *sheng* (each time) and three times a day.

【今译】

使用发汗法以后,致使患者腹部胀满的,宜用厚朴生姜半夏甘草人参汤治疗。

【原文】

(六七)

伤寒,若吐若下后,心下逆满,气上冲胸,起则头眩,脉沉紧,发汗则动经,身为振振摇者,茯苓桂枝白术甘草汤主之。

茯苓桂枝白术甘草汤

茯苓四两、桂枝三两(去皮)、白术二两、甘草二两(炙)。

右四味,以水六升,煮取三升,取滓,分温三服。

【今译】

伤寒病中,患者或经过涌吐法或经过攻下法治疗以后,感觉心下气逆闷满,气上冲胸膈,头晕目眩,脉象沉紧,再用汗法会影响经脉,使身体振振颤动,宜用苓桂术甘汤治疗。

【原文】

(六八)

发汗,病不解,反恶寒者,虚故也。芍药甘草附子汤主之。

Differentiation of pulse and syndrome/pattern
[*related to*] *taiyang disease and treatment* (*part 2*)

【英译】

Line 67

[The disease caused by] cold damage [is characterized by] either vomiting or diarrhea, fullness underneath the heart and counterflow of qi in the chest, [consequently causing] dizziness, deep and tight pulse, diaphoresis that affects meridians and vibration of the body. [It] can be treated by Fuling Guizhi Baizhu Gancao Decoction (茯苓桂枝白术甘草汤, poria, cinnamon twig, ovate atractylodes and licorice decoction).

Fuling Guizhi Baizhu Gancao Decoction (茯苓桂枝白术甘草汤, poria, cinnamon twig, ovate atractylodes and licorice decoction) [is composed of] 4 *liang* of Fuling (茯苓, poria, Poria), 3 *liang* of Guizhi (桂枝, cinnamon twig, Ramulus Cinnamomi) (bark-removed), 2 *liang* of Baizhu (白术, rhizome of largehead atractylodes, Rhizoma Atractylodis Macrocephalae) and 2 *liang* of Gancao (甘草, licorice, Radix Glycyrrhizae Praeparata) (broiled).

These four ingredients are decocted in 6 *sheng* of water to get 3 *sheng* [after] boiling. The dregs are removed and [the decoction is] taken warm 1 *sheng* [each time] and three times a day.

【英译】

Line 68

Failure of diaphoresis to relieve the disease with aversion to cold is due to deficiency. [It can be] treated by Shaoyao Gancao Fuzi Decoction (芍药甘草附子汤, peony, licorice and aconite decoction).

芍药甘草附子汤方

芍药、甘草各三两(炙)、附子一枚(炮,去皮,破八片)。

右三味,以水五升,煮取一升五合,去滓,分温三服。

【今译】

使用发汗法治疗后,患者病未解除,反而恶寒,这是虚弱所致,宜用芍药甘草附子汤治疗。

【原文】

(六九)

发汗,若下之,病仍不解,烦躁者,茯苓四逆汤主之。

茯苓四逆汤方

茯苓六两、人参一两、附子一枚(生用,去皮,破八片)、甘草二两(炙)、干姜一两半。

右五味,以水五升,煮取三升,去滓,温服七合,日三服。

【今译】

使用发汗法,或泻下法以后,患者病请仍未解除,却出现了烦躁不安等症的,宜用茯苓四逆汤治疗。

Differentiation of pulse and syndrome/pattern [related to] taiyang disease and treatment（part 2）

Shaoyao Gancao Fuzi Decoction（芍药甘草附子汤，peony, licorice and aconite decoction）[is composed of] 3 *liang* of Shaoyao（芍药，peony，Radix Paeoniae），3 *liang* of Gancao（甘草，licorice，Radix Glycyrrhizae Praeparata）（broiled）and 1 piece of Fuzi（附子，aconite，Radix Aconiti Lateralis Preparata）（fry heavily，remove peel，pound into eight small pieces）.

These three ingredients are decocted in 5 *sheng* of water to get 1.5 *sheng* [after] boiling. The dregs are removed and [the decoction is] taken warm 1 *sheng* [each time] and three times a day.

【英译】

Line 69

[If] the disease is not relieved after diaphoresis or even after purgation [with] dysphoria，[it can be] treated by Fuling Sini Decoction（茯苓四逆汤，poria decoction for resolving four kinds of adverseness）.

Fuling Sini Decoction（茯苓四逆汤，poria decoction for resolving four kinds of adverseness）[is composed of] 4 *liang* of Fuling（茯苓，poria，Poria），1 *liang* of Renshen（人参，ginseng，Radix Ginseng），1 piece of Fuzi（附子，aconite，Radix Aconiti Lateralis Preparata）[rough，to be broken into eight small pieces with peel removed]，2 *liang* of Gancao（甘草，licorice，Radix Glycyrrhizae Praeparata）（broiled）and 1.5 *liang* of Ganjiang（干姜，dried ginger，Rhizoma Zingiberis）.

These five ingredients are decocted in 5 *sheng* of water to get 3 *sheng* [after] boiling. The dregs are removed and [the decoction is] taken warm 7 *ge* [each time] and thrice a day.

【原文】

（七〇）

发汗后，恶寒者，虚故也。不恶寒，但热者，实也。当和胃气，与调胃承气汤。

【今译】

发汗后有恶寒表现的，是气虚所致；不恶寒的，但见发热，为邪气盛实所致，应当调和胃气，宜用调胃承气汤治疗。

【原文】

（七一）

太阳病，发汗后，大汗出，胃中干，烦躁不得眠，欲得饮水者，少少与饮之，令胃气和则愈。若脉浮，小便不利，微热消渴者，五苓散主之。

五苓散方

猪苓十八铢（去皮）、泽泻一两六铢半、白术十八铢、茯苓十八铢、桂枝半两（去皮）。

右五味，捣为散，以白饮和服方寸匕，日三服，多饮暖水，汗出愈，如法将息。

【今译】

太阳病，使用发汗法后，导致大量流汗，胃中津液不足，使患者烦躁不安，不能安眠。口干想喝水的，可喝少量的水，使胃气调和，病就可愈。若脉象浮，小便不畅，有微热，渴饮不止，宜用五苓散治疗。

Differentiation of pulse and syndrome / pattern [related to] taiyang disease and treatment (part 2)

【英译】

Line 70

Aversion to cold after perspiration is due to deficiency. [If there is] no aversion to cold [but] fever, [it is due to] excess. To harmonize stomach qi, Tiaowei Chengqi Decoction (调胃承气汤, decoction for regulating the stomach and harmonizing qi) [should be used].

【英译】

Line 71

[The patient with] taiyang disease, [characterized by] profuse sweating after inducing perspiration, dryness in the stomach and insomnia due to dysphoria, should drink a little water in order to harmonize stomach qi and heal [the disease]. If [there are symptoms and signs of] floating pulse, dysuria, slight fever and wasting-thirst, Wuling Powder (五苓散, powder made of five medicinal herbs) [can be used] to treat [it].

Wuling Powder (五苓散, powder made of five medicinal herbs) [is composed of] 18 *zhu* of Zhuling (猪苓, polyporus, Polyporus Umbellatus) with peel removed, 1 *liang* and 6.5 *zhu* of Zexie (泽泻, alisma, Rhizoma Alismatis), 18 *zhu* of Baizhu (白术, rhizome of largeheade atractylodes, Rhizoma Atractylodis Macrocephalae), 18 *zhu* of Fuling (茯苓, poria, Poria) and 0.5 *liang* of Guizhi (桂枝, cinnamon twig, Ramulus Cinnamomi) with bark removed.

These five ingredients are pounded into powder [which is] mixed with rice soup. [The decoction is] taken with a square spoon three times a day. [Besides, the patient should] drink more warm water. [When] sweating occurs, [the disease will] heal. The method [for regulation and healthcare is] the same [as that for using Guizhi Decoction (桂枝汤, cinnamon twig decoction)].

【原文】

(七二)

发汗已,脉浮数,烦渴者,五苓散主之。

【今译】

使用发汗法之后,患者脉象浮数,烦躁口渴的,宜用五苓散主治。

【原文】

(七三)

伤寒,汗出而渴者,五苓散主之;不渴者,茯苓甘草汤主之。

茯苓甘草汤方

茯苓二两,桂枝二两去皮,甘草一两,炙生姜三两,切片以上四味药,用水四升,煎煮成二升,去掉药渣,分成三次温服。

【今译】

伤寒病,出汗而口渴的,可用五苓散治疗;口不渴的,可用茯苓甘草汤治疗。

Differentiation of pulse and syndrome / pattern [*related to*] *taiyang disease and treatment* (*part 2*)

【英译】

Line 72

[The disease, characterized by] floating and rapid pulse, dysphoria and thirst after diaphoresis, [can be] treated by Wuling Powder (五苓散, powder made of five medicinal herbs).

【英译】

Line 73

[The disease caused by] cold damage, [characterized by] sweating and thirst, [can be] treated by Wuling Powder (五苓散, powder made of five medicinal herbs). [If there is] no thirst, [it can be] treated by Fuling Gancao Decoction (茯苓甘草汤, poria and licorice decoction).

Fuling Gancao Decoction (茯苓甘草汤, poria and licorice decoction) [is composed of] 2 *liang* of Fuling (茯苓, poria, Poria), 2 *liang* of Guizhi (桂枝, cinnamon twig, Ramulus Cinnamomi) with bark removed, 1 *liang* of Gancao (甘草, licorice, Radix Glycyrrhizae Praeparata) and 3 *liang* of Shengjiang (生姜, fresh ginger, Rhizoma Zingiberis Recens) broiled and cut.

These four ingredients are decocted in 4 *sheng* of water to get 2 *sheng* [after] boiling. The dregs are removed and [the decoction is] taken warm for three times.

【原文】

(七四)

中风发热,六七日不解而烦,有表里证,渴欲饮水,水入则吐者,名曰水逆,五苓散主之。

【今译】

中风发热,六七天后还未解除,使患者烦闷,有表里之证。若有口渴想喝水,而喝水即呕吐等症状,名为水逆,宜用五苓散主治。

【原文】

(七五)

未持脉时,病人手叉自冒心。师因教试令咳而不咳者,此必两耳聋无闻也。所以然者,以重发汗,虚故如此。发汗后,饮水多必喘,以水灌之亦喘。

【今译】

医生未诊脉时,病人双手交叉按压心胸。如果医生让病人咳嗽,病人却没有任何反应,说明病人双耳失去了听力。之所以如此,是因为多汗致虚的缘故。发汗后,饮水太多必然喘咳,甚至用水洗身,也会引起咳喘。

Differentiation of pulse and syndrome/pattern [related to] taiyang disease and treatment（part 2）

【英译】

Line 74

Wind stroke with fever，[which is] not relieved after six or seven days，[characterized by] external and internal syndrome/pattern and vomiting after drinking water with desire to drink water，is called counterflow of water. [It can be] treated by Wuling Powder（五苓散，powder made of five medicinal herbs）.

【英译】

Line 75

Before taking the pulse，the patient presses the chest with folded hands. [If] there is no response [when] the doctor asks [the patient] to cough，[it indicates that the patient] must be deaf due to heavy and profuse sweating [which causes] deficiency. After perspiration，[the patient will] pant after drinking more water or washing the body.

【原文】

（七六）

发汗后,水药不得入口为逆。若更发汗,必吐下不止。发汗吐下后,虚烦不得眠,若剧者,必反复颠倒,心中懊恼,栀子豉汤主之。若少气者,栀子甘草豉汤主之;若呕者,栀子生姜豉汤主之。

栀子豉汤方

栀子十四枚(掰,味甘寒)、香豉四合(绵裹,味苦寒)。

上二味,以水四升,先煮栀子,得二升半,内豉,煮取一升半,去滓,分为二服,温进一服。得吐者,止后服。

【今译】

如果发汗之后,患者无法服药和饮水,是逆证。如果再次发汗,必然导致呕吐和腹泻不止。发汗而引起的呕吐和腹泻后,患者还有虚烦和睡不着的症状。如果病情再剧烈,患者必然翻来覆去,心中烦乱,可用栀子豉汤主治。如果少气,可用栀子甘草豉汤主治;如果呕吐,可用栀子生姜豉汤主治。

Differentiation of pulse and syndrome / pattern [related to] taiyang disease and treatment (part 2)

【英译】

Line 76

After perspiration [induced], [the patient] cannot take water or medicine, [it is an] adverse [case]. If perspiration [is induced] again, [the patient] must [suffer from] repeated vomiting and diarrhea, [consequently leading to] dysphoria due to deficiency and insomnia. If severe, [the patient] will tumble [on the bed, feeling] vexed, [which can be] treated by Zhizi Chi Decoction (栀子豉汤, gardenia and fermented soybean decoction). If [there is] shortness of breath, Zhizi Gancao Chi Decoction (栀子甘草豉汤, gardenia, licorice and fermented soybean decoction)[can be] used. If [there is] vomiting, Zhizi Shengjiang Chi Decoction (栀子生姜豉汤, gardenia, ginger and fermented soybean decoction)[can be] used.

Zhizi Chi Decoction (栀子豉汤, gardenia and fermented soybean decoction) [is composed of] 14 pieces of Zhizi (栀子, gardenia, Fructus Gardeniae) (broken, sweet in taste and cold in property)and 4 *ge* of Xiangchi (香豉, fermented soybean, Semen Sojae Praeparatum) wrapped in cotton gauze, bitter in taste and cold in property.

These two ingredients are decocted in 4 *sheng* of water. Zhizi (栀子, gardenia, Fructus Gardeniae) is decocted first to reduce 2.5 *sheng* [of water]. [Then] Xiangchi (香豉, fermented soybean, Semen Sojae Praeparatum) is decocted to get 1.5 *sheng* [after] boiling. The dregs are removed and [the decoction is] divided into two doses [to be] taken warm [one each time]. [If there is] vomiting, rest [of the decoction] should not be taken.

【原文】

(七七)

发汗,若下之,而烦热,胸中窒者,栀子豉汤主之。

【今译】

发汗过后,如果再用泻下法,则会出现心胸烦热,胸中窒塞等症状,可用栀子豉汤主治。

【原文】

(七八)

伤寒五六日,大下之后,身热不去,心中结痛者,未欲解也。栀子豉汤主之。

【今译】

外感病发作五六日后,使用了大剂量的泻下药,但身热却未退,患者感到心胸结塞疼痛,这是病未解除的缘故,宜用栀子豉汤治疗。

【原文】

(七九)

伤寒下后,心烦,腹满,卧起不安者,栀子厚朴汤主之。

Differentiation of pulse and syndrome/pattern [related to] taiyang disease and treatment (part 2)

【英译】

Line 77

[After application of] diaphoresis or purgation, [there are still symptoms and signs of] dysphoria, fever and suffocation, Zhizi Chi Decoction (栀子豉汤, gardenia and fermented soybean decoction) [can be used] to treat it.

【英译】

Line 78

Five to six days [after occurrence of] cold damage, [if there are still symptoms and signs of] constant fever, suffocation and pain in the chest after [application of] drastic purgation, [it can be] treated by Zhizi Chi Decoction (栀子豉汤, gardenia and fermented soybean decoction).

【英译】

Line 79

After [application of] purgation [for treating] cold damage, [if there are still symptoms and signs of] dysphoria, abdominal fullness and restlessness [when] lying on bed or getting up, [it can be] treated by Zhizi Houpo Decoction (栀子厚朴汤, gardenia and magnolia bark decoction).

Zhizi Houpo Decoction (栀子厚朴汤, gardenia and magnolia bark decoction) [is composed of] 15 pieces of Zhizi (栀子, gardenia, Fructus Gardeniae) to be broken, 4 *liang* of Houpo (厚

栀子厚朴汤方

栀子十四个(擘)、厚朴四两(炙,去皮)、枳实四枚(水浸,炙令黄)。

右三味,以水三升半,煮取一升半,去滓,分两服,温进一服,得吐者,止后服。

【今译】

外感病,使用泻下法治疗之后,患者有心烦不宁、腹部胀满、坐卧不安等症状,宜用栀子厚朴汤主治。

【原文】

(八〇)

伤寒,医以丸药大下之,身热不去,微烦者,栀子干姜汤主之。

栀子干姜汤方

栀子十四个(擘)、干姜二两。

右二味,以水三升半,煮取一升半,去滓,分两服,温进一服,得吐者,止后服。

【今译】

伤寒病,医生若用泻下丸药攻下,就会出现身热不退,微烦不安,宜用栀子干姜汤主治。

Differentiation of pulse and syndrome / pattern [related to] taiyang disease and treatment (part 2)

朴， magnolia bark，Cortex Magnoliae Officinalis) with bark removed and broiled and 4 pieces of Zhishi (枳实，processed unripe bitter orange，Fructus Aurantii Immaturus) to be soaked in water and broiled yellow.

These three ingredients are decocted in 3. 5 *sheng* of water to get 1. 5 *sheng* [after] boiling. The dregs are removed and [the decoction is] divided into two doses to be taken warm one [each time]. [If] there is vomiting, rest [of the decoction should] not be taken.

【英译】

Line 80

[When] cold damage [is treated by] drastic purgation with pills，[there are still] constant fever and moderate dysphoria，Zhizi Ganjiang Decoction （栀子干姜汤，gardenia and dry ginger decoction） [can be used to] treat it.

Zhizi Ganjiang Decoction （栀子干姜汤，gardenia and dry ginger decoction） [is composed of] 14 pieces of Zhizi （栀子，gardenia，Fructus Gardeniae）(broken) and 2 *liang* of Ganjiang（干姜，dried ginger，Rhizoma Zingiberis）.

These two ingredients are decocted in 3 *sheng* of water to get 1. 5 *sheng* [after] boiling. The dregs are removed and [the decoction is] divided into two doses to be taken warm one [each time]. [If] there is vomiting, rest [of the decoction should] not be taken.

【原文】

(八一)

凡用栀子汤,病人旧微溏者,不可与服之。

【今译】

凡用栀子豉汤时,如果病人平素大便稀溏,不可使用。

【原文】

(八二)

太阳病,发汗,汗出不解,其人仍发热,心下悸,头眩,身𰀓动,振振欲擗地者,真武汤主之。

真武汤方

茯苓三两、芍药三两、白术二两、生姜三两(切)、附子一枚(炮,去皮,破八片)。

右五味,以水八升,煮取三升,去滓,温服七合,日三服。若咳者,加五味子半升,细辛一两,干姜一两。若小便利者,去茯苓。若下利者,去芍药,加干姜二两。若呕者,去附子,加生姜,足前为半斤。

【今译】

太阳病,使用发汗法后,虽然出汗了,但病却未解,患者仍然发热,心悸,头晕目眩,全身肌肉颤动,身体震颤像要跌倒似的,宜用真武汤主治。

Differentiation of pulse and syndrome / pattern
[related to] taiyang disease and treatment (part 2)

【英译】

Line 81

Zhizi Decoction (栀子汤, gardenia decoction) cannot be used [to treat] patients with frequent sloppy stool.

【英译】

Line 82

[When treated by] diaphoresis, [the patient with] taiyang disease is not cured, still [suffering from] fever, palpitation, dizziness, vibration and shivering. [It can be] treated by Zhenwu Decoction (真武汤, true warrior decoction).

Zhenwu Decoction (真武汤, true warrior decoction) [is composed of] 3 *liang* of Fuling (茯苓, poria, Poria), 3 *liang* of Shaoyao (芍药, peony, Radix Paeoniae), 2 *liang* of Baizhu (白术, rhizome of largehead atractylodes, Rhizoma Atractylodis Macrocephalae), 3 *liang* of Shengjiang (生姜, fresh ginger, Rhizoma Zingiberis Recens) (cut) and 1 piece of Fuzi (附子, aconite, Radix Aconiti Lateralis Preparata) (fried heavily, remove the peel and break into eight small pieces).

These five ingredients are decocted in 8 *sheng* of water to get 3 *sheng* [after] boiling. The dregs are removed and [the decoction is] taken warm 7 *ge* [each time] and three times a day. If [there is] cough, 0.5 *sheng* of Wuweizi (五味子, schisandra, Fructus Schisandrae), 1 *liang* of Xixin (细辛, asarum, Herba Asari) and 1 *liang* of Ganjiang (干姜, dried ginger, Rhizoma Zingiberis) are added. If urination is uninhibited, Fuling (茯苓, poria, Poria) [should be] removed. If [there is] diarrhea, Shaoyao (芍药, peony, Radix Paeoniae) is removed and 2 *liang* of Ganjiang (干姜, dried ginger, Rhizoma Zingiberis) is added. If [there is] retching, Fuzi (附子, aconite, Radix Aconiti Lateralis Preparata) is removed and Shengjiang (生姜, fresh ginger, Rhizoma Zingiberis Recens) is added to 0.5 *jin*.

【原文】

(八三)

咽喉干燥者,不可发汗。

【今译】

咽喉干燥的,不可用发汗法。

【原文】

(八四)

淋家,不可发汗,发汗必便血。

【今译】

患淋病的病人,不能用发汗法治疗,误用发汗法必然会导致便血。

【原文】

(八五)

疮家,虽身疼痛,不可发汗,汗出则痉。

【今译】

患有疮疡的病人,虽然身体疼痛,但也不可用发汗法治疗。误用发汗法,就会导致筋脉强急。

Differentiation of pulse and syndrome / pattern [related to] taiyang disease and treatment (part 2)

【英译】

Line 83

[The patient suffering from] dryness of throat cannot [be treated by] diaphoresis.

【英译】

Line 84

[Patient with] urinary dripping cannot [be treated by] diaphoresis, [otherwise] hematuria will be caused.

【英译】

Line 85

[Patient with] sores, although [suffering from] generalized pain, cannot [be treated by] diaphoresis, [otherwise] tetany will be caused.

【原文】

(八六)

衄家,不可发汗,汗出必额上陷,脉急紧,直视不能眴,不得眠。

【今译】

衄血的病人,不可用发汗法治疗。误用发汗法,就会出现额部上陷处脉急紧,两眼直视而不能转动,无法睡眠等病变。

【原文】

(八七)

亡血家,不可发汗,发汗则寒栗而振。

【今译】

有失血的病人,不可使用发汗法治疗。误用发汗法,就会引发寒栗、震颤等症状。

【原文】

(八八)

汗家,重发汗,必恍惚心乱,小便已,阴疼,与禹余粮丸。

禹余粮丸方

因历史原因,禹余粮丸方未见《伤寒论》。据 992 年出版的《太平圣惠方》,在 960—1279 年间的宋朝,禹余粮丸方构成如下:

龙骨、紫石英各 30 克,人参、桂心、川乌头各 15 克,泽泻、桑寄生、石斛、当归、杜仲、肉苁蓉各 30 克,远志、五味子、甘草各 15 克

Differentiation of pulse and syndrome/pattern [related to] taiyang disease and treatment（part 2）

【英译】

Line 86

[Patient with] epistaxis cannot [be treated by] diaphoresis，[otherwise] it will cause tension of vessels in the depressions of forehead，difficulty in moving the eyes and insomnia.

【英译】

Line 87

[Patient with] hemorrhage cannot [be treated by] diaphoresis，[otherwise] it will cause chilliness and quivering.

【英译】

Line 88

[Patient with] frequent sweating [treated by] diaphoresis will [suffer from] derangement and urodynia after urination. [It can be] treated by Yuyuliang Pill（禹余粮丸，limonite pill）.

Note：

Due to historical reasons，the composition of Yuyuliang Pill（禹余粮丸，limonite pill）cannot be found in *On Cold Damage*（《伤寒论》）. According to *Taiping Shenghui Formulae*（《太平圣惠方》）published in 992 A. D. in the Song Dynasty（960 A. D.—1279 A. D.），this Yuyuliang Decoction（禹余粮丸，limonite pill）[is composed of] 30 - 60g of Yuyuliang（禹余粮，limonite，Limonitum），30g of Longgu（龙骨，loong bone，Os Loong），30g of Zishiying（紫石英，fluorite，Fluoritum），15g of Renshen（人参，

【今译】

　　常出汗的患者,若再用发汗法治疗,就会引发心神恍惚、慌乱不宁,小便后尿道疼痛等症状,用禹余粮丸治疗。

【原文】

　　(八九)

　　病人有寒,复发汗,胃中冷,必吐蛕。

【今译】

　　有内寒的病人,不能再用发汗法治疗。如果再用发汗法治疗,必然导致胃冷及吐蛔等症状的出现。

【原文】

　　(九〇)

　　本发汗,而复下之,此为逆也。若先发汗,治不为逆。本先下之,而反汗之,为逆。若先下之,治不为逆。

【今译】

　　本来应该发汗治疗,反而采用攻下法治疗,这是误用。如果先发汗解表,就不会造成误治。本来应该先用攻下法治疗,反而使用了发汗法治疗,也是误治。如果先用攻下法治疗,治法上就不会出现失误。

Differentiation of pulse and syndrome / pattern [related to] taiyang disease and treatment (part 2)

ginseng, Radix Ginseng), 15g of Guixin（桂心, cinnamon cortex, Cortex Cinnamomi）, 15g of Chuanwutou（川乌头, aconite root, Radix Aconiti）, 30g of Zexie（泽泻, alisma, Rhizoma Alismatis）, 30g of Sangjisheng（桑寄生, parasitic loranthus, Herba Taxilli）, 30g of Shihu（石斛, dendrobe, Herba Dendrobii）, 30g of Danggui（当归, Chinese angelica, Radix Angelicae Sinensis）, 30g of Duzhong（杜仲, eucommia bark, Cortex Eucommiae）, 30g of Roucongrong（肉苁蓉, desertliving cistanche, Herba Cistanches）, 15g of Yuanzhi（远志, polygala root, Radix Polygalae）, 15g Wuweizi（五味子, fruit of Chinese magnoliavine, Fructus Schisandrae）and 15g of Gancao（甘草, licorice, Radix Glycyrrhizae Praeparata）.

【英译】

Line 89

The patient with cold [treated by] diaphoresis [will feel] chilly in the stomach and vomit rounworms.

【英译】

Line 90

[Cold damage] should [be treated by] diaphoresis. [If it is treated by] purgation, it is a wrong [treatment]. If perspiration is promoted first, [it is] not an incorrect [treatment]. Originally [it should be treated by] purgation first [and then by diaphoresis]. [If treated by] diaphoresis first, [it is] a wrong [treatment]. [If treated by] purgation first, [it is] not a wrong [treatment].

【原文】

（九一）

伤寒，医下之，续得下利，清谷不止，身疼痛者，急当救里；后身疼痛，清便自调者，急当救表。救里宜四逆汤，救表宜桂枝汤。

【今译】

伤寒病，医生如果用泻下法治疗，会使病人继续下利清谷不止，身体疼痛，此时应当急除里邪。祛除里邪之后，患者身体依然疼痛，但大便恢复正常，此时应当急除表邪。祛除里邪宜用四逆汤，祛除表邪宜用桂枝汤。

【原文】

（九二）

病发热，头痛，脉反沉，若不差，身体疼痛，当救其里，宜四逆汤。

【今译】

病人发热，头痛，脉反而沉。如果病人症状不解，身体疼痛，应当治里，宜用四逆汤方治疗。

Differentiation of pulse and syndrome / pattern
[related to] taiyang disease and treatment (part 2)

【英译】

Line 91

[If] cold damage [disease is treated by] purgation, [it will] result in diarrhea with undigested food and generalized pain, [which] should [be treated by] relieving the internal. After [treatment, if there is still] generalized pain and defecation is regulated spontaneously, [it] should [be treated by] relieving the external. To relieve the internal, Sini Decoction (四逆汤, decoction for resolving four kinds of adverseness) should [be used]; to relieve the external, Guizhi Decoction (桂枝汤, cinnamon twig decoction) should [be used].

【英译】

Line 92

[When the patient] suffers from fever, headache and deep pulse, [if the disease is] not healed [after treatment and there is still] generalized pain, the internal should be relieved by Sini Decoction (四逆汤, decoction for resolving four kinds of adverseness).

【原文】

(九三)

太阳病,先下之而不愈,因复发汗,以此表里俱虚,其人因致冒。冒家汗出自愈。所以然者,汗出表和故也。里未和,然后复下之。

【今译】

太阳病,先用泻下法治疗而未痊愈,再用发汗法治疗,导致内外皆虚,使得患者有头晕昏沉症状。头晕昏沉的患者如果能出汗,就可自行痊愈。之所以如此,是因为汗出后表气能得以调和的原因。若里气尚未调和,然后再用泻下法予以治疗。

【原文】

(九四)

太阳病,未解,脉阴阳俱停,必先振栗,汗出而解。但阳脉微者,先汗出而解;但阴脉微者,下之而解。若欲下之,宜调胃承气汤。

【今译】

太阳病,尚未解除时,阴阳脉突然停止搏动,必然首先引起战栗,然后汗出而病解。如果阳脉(即独寸)开始搏动,先出汗而后病解;如果阴脉(即尺脉)微微搏动的,泻下后而病解。如要使用泻下法,宜用调胃承气汤。

Differentiation of pulse and syndrome / pattern [related to] taiyang disease and treatment (part 2)

【英译】

Line 93

[If] taiyang disease [is treated] first by purgation and is not healed, [it is then treated] again by diaphoresis, resulting in dual deficiency of the external and internal, and causing dizziness. [If the patient with] dizziness perspires, [the disease will] heal spontaneously. The reason [is that] perspiration harmonizes the external. [If] the internal is not harmonized, purgation can be used again.

【英译】

Line 94

[If] taiyang disease is not healed, both yin pulse (at the chi region) and yang pulse (at the cun region) are deepened, causing shivering and chilliness [which can be] relieved by perspiration. [If] yang pulse is felt feeble, perspiration [should be] induced first to relieve [it]. [If] yin pulse is felt feeble, purgation [should be used] to relieve [it]. For the purpose of purgation, Tiaowei Chengqi Decoction (调胃承气汤, deccoction for regulating the stomach and harmonizing qi) should be used.

【原文】

(九五)

太阳病,发热、汗出者,此为营弱卫强,故使汗出。欲救邪风者,宜桂枝汤。

【今译】

太阳病,发热出汗的,即营阴弱不能内守,卫气盛而与邪相争所致,治疗须驱风散邪,宜用桂枝汤主治。

【原文】

(九六)

伤寒五六日,中风,往来寒热,胸胁苦满,嘿嘿不欲饮食,心烦喜呕,或胸中烦而不呕,或渴,或腹中痛,或胁下痞鞕,或心下悸、小便不利,或不渴、身有微热,或咳者,小柴胡汤主之。

小柴胡汤方

柴胡半斤(味苦,微寒)、黄芩三两(味苦寒)、人参三两(味甘温)、甘草三两(味甘平)、半夏半升(洗,味辛温)、生姜三两(切,味辛温)、大枣

Differentiation of pulse and syndrome / pattern [related to] taiyang disease and treatment (part 2)

【英译】

Line 95

Taiyang disease [characterized by] fever and perspiration indicates that nutrient qi is weak while defense qi is strong. That is why [there is] perspiration. The appropriate [formula for treating it is] Guizhi Decoction (桂枝汤, cinnamon twig decoction).

【英译】

Line 96

Cold damage [disease], five to six days [after occurrence], [characterized by] wind stroke, intermittent chilliness and fever, thoracic and costal fullness and discomfort, no desire to speak, reluctance in drinking water and taking food, dysphoria, frequent nausea, or thoracic restlessness without nausea, or thirst, or abdominal pain, or lump below the costal region, or palpitation and dysuria, or no thirst and slight fever, or cough, [can be] treated by Xiao Chaihu Decoction (小柴胡汤, minor bupleurum decoction).

Xiao Chaihu Decoction (小柴胡汤, minor bupleurum decoction) [is composed of] 0.5 *jin* of Chaihu (柴胡, bupleurum, Radix Bupleuri) bitter in taste and slight cold in property, 3 *liang* of Huangqin (黄芩, scutellaria, Radix Scutellariae) bitter in taste and cold in property, 3 *liang* of Renshen (人参, ginseng, Radix Ginseng) sweet in taste and warm in property, 3 *liang* of Gancao (甘草, licorice, Radix Glycyrrhizae Praeparata) sweet in taste and bland in property, 0.5 *sheng* of Banxia (半夏, pinellia, Rhizoma Pinelliae) washed, pungent in taste and warm in property, 3 *liang* of Shengjiang (生姜, fresh ginger,

十二枚(掰,味甘温)。

右七味,以水一斗二升,煮取六升,去滓,再煎,取三升,温服一升,日三服。

后加减法:

若胸中烦而不呕,去半夏、人参,加栝蒌实一枚。

若渴者,去半夏,加人参,合前成四两半,栝蒌根四两。

若腹中痛者,去黄芩,加芍药三两。

若胁下痞鞕,去大枣,加牡蛎四两。

若心下悸,小便不利者,去黄芩,加茯苓四两。

若不渴,外有微热者,去人参,加桂三两,温覆取微汗愈。

若咳者,去人参、大枣、生姜,加五味子半升,干姜二两。

【今译】

伤寒病发作五六日后中风,出现寒来热往,胸胁苦满,静默不语,不思饮食,时而心烦喜呕。或胸中烦闷但却不呕吐,或口中作渴,或腹中疼痛,或胁下痞塞硬满,或心悸而小便不利,或口不渴而体表微热,或有咳嗽,均宜用小柴胡汤治疗。

Differentiation of pulse and syndrome / pattern [related to] taiyang disease and treatment（part 2）

Rhizoma Zingiberis Recens）cut，pangent in taste and warm in property，and 12 pieces of Dazao（大枣，jujube，Fructus Ziziphus Jujubae）broken sweet in taste and warm in property.

These seven ingredients are decocted in 1 *dou* and 2 *sheng* of water to get 6 *sheng* [after] boiling. The dregs are removed and [it is] decocted again to get 3 *sheng* [after] boiling. [The final decoction] is taken warm 1 *sheng* [each time] and three times a day.

Modifications [of the decoction]：

If there is thoracic dysphoria without nausea，remove Banxia （半夏，pinellia，Rhizoma Pinelliae）and Renshen（人参，ginseng，Radix Ginseng）and add 1 piece of Gualoushi（栝蒌实，trichosanthes semen，Fructus Trichosanthis）.

If there is thirst，remove Banxia （半夏，pinellia，Rhizoma Pinelliae）and add Renshen（人参，ginseng，Radix Ginseng），increasing it to 4 *liang* with the original quota，and 4 *liang* of Gualougen（栝蒌根，trichosanthes root，Radix Trichosanthis）.

If there is abdominal pain，remove Huangqin （黄芩，scutellaria，Radix Scutellariae）and add 3 *liang* of Shaoyao（芍药，peony，Radix Paeoniae）.

If there is lump below the costal region，remove Dazao（大枣，jujube，Fructus Ziziphus Jujubae）and add 4 *liang* of Muli（牡蛎，oyster shell，Concha Ostreae）.

If there is palpitation and dysuria，remove Huangqin（黄芩，scutellaria，Radix Scutellariae）and add 4 *liang* of Fuling（茯苓，poria，Poria）.

If there is no thirst but slight external fever，remove Renshen （人参，ginseng，Radix Ginseng）and add 3 *liang* of Guizhi（桂枝，

【原文】

(九七)

血弱气尽,腠理开,邪气因入,与正气相搏,结于胁下,正邪分争,往来寒热,休作有时,嘿嘿不欲饮食,脏腑相连,其痛必下,邪高痛下,故使呕也,小柴胡汤主之。服柴胡汤已,渴者属阳明,以法治之。

【今译】

血虚弱而气耗尽,腠理豁开,邪气乘虚而入,与正气相搏结,留结于胁下,正气与邪气争搏,引发寒热往来,时有停止,时有发作,使患者表情沉默、不思饮食。由于脏腑相连,必然出现腹痛。由于邪气在上,痛在腹下,因此出现呕吐,宜用小柴胡汤治疗。服用小柴胡汤后,出现口渴欲饮现象的属阳明证,须按阳明证治法进行治疗。

Differentiation of pulse and syndrome/pattern [related to] taiyang disease and treatment (part 2)

cinnamon twig, Ramulus Cinnamomi). [Ask the patient to put on more clothes or to cover with a quilt. If the patient feels] warm and begins to sweat, [it is helpful for] healing [the disease].

If there is cough, remove Renshen (人 参, ginseng, Radix Ginseng), Dazao (大 枣, jujube, Fructus Ziziphus Jujubae) and Shengjiang (生姜, fresh ginger, Rhizoma Zingiberis Recens), add 0.5 *jin* Wuweizi (五味子, Chinese magnoliavine, Fructus Schisandrae) and 2 *liang* of Ganjiang (干姜, dried ginger, Rhizoma Zingiberis).

【英译】

Line 97

[The disease is characterized by] weakness of blood, deficiency of qi, looseness of interstices, invasion of pathogenic factors that struggle with healthy qi and binds beneath the costal region, conflict between pathogenic factors and healthy qi, intermittent chilliness and fever at certain intervals, no desire to speak, reluctance in drinking water and taking food, abdominal pain due to interaction between zang-organs and fu-organs and causing nausea. [It can be] treated by Xiao Chaihu Decoction (小柴胡汤, minor bupleurum decoction). [If there is] thirst [after] taking [Xiao] Chaihu Decoction (小柴胡汤, minor bupleurum decoction), [it shows that the disease is already] transmitted to yangming [and should be] treated with the therapeutic methods [used to treat yangming syndrome/pattern].

【原文】

(九八)

得病六七日,脉迟浮弱,恶风寒,手足温,医二三下之,不能食而胁下满痛,面目及身黄,颈项强,小便难者,与柴胡汤,后必下重。本渴饮水而呕者,柴胡汤不中与也,食谷者哕。

【今译】

得病六七日后,患者脉搏迟而浮,恶风寒,手足温暖。医生曾用泻下法治疗两三次,但患者出现了不能饮食,胁下胀满而疼痛,面部、眼睛和周身均发黄,颈项强拘,小便困难等症状。以柴胡汤主治,必使患者大便时肛部有下坠之感。本来口渴饮水而呕的,或进食后有呃逆的,均不宜于用柴胡汤治疗。

【原文】

(九九)

伤寒四五日,身热,恶风,颈项强,胁下满,手足温而渴者,小柴胡汤主之。

【今译】

外感病发作四五天后,患者身体发热,恶风,颈项拘急,胁下胀满,手足温暖而又口渴的,宜用小柴胡汤主治。

Differentiation of pulse and syndrome / pattern [related to] taiyang disease and treatment (part 2)

【英译】

Line 98

[The disease], six or seven days [after occurrence], [is characterized by] slow, floating and weak pulse, aversion to wind and cold, and warmth of hands and feet. [If] the doctor [has used] purgation [to treat] it for two or three times, [it will result in] difficulty in taking food, fullness and pain beneath the costal region, yellow face, eyes and body and dysuria. [If] Chaihu Decoction (柴胡汤, bupleurum decoction) [is used to treat it], [it will lead to] anal tenesmus. Originally [there is] thirst, [but there will be] vomiting [after] drinking water. [To treat such a disease,] Chaihu Decoction (柴胡汤, bupleurum decoction) cannot be used, [otherwise] nausea [will be caused after] taking food.

【英译】

Line 99

Cold damage [disease], four to five days [after occurrence], [is characterized by] fever, aversion to wind, stiffness of neck and nape, fullness beneath the costal region, warmth of hands and feet, and thirst. [It can be] treated by Xiao Chaihu Decoction (小柴胡汤, minor bupleurum decoction).

【原文】

(一○○)

伤寒,阳脉涩,阴脉弦,法当腹中急痛,先与小建中汤;不差者,小柴胡汤主之。

小建中汤方

桂枝三两(去皮,味辛热)、甘草三两(炙,味甘平)、大枣十二枚(掰,味甘温)、芍药六两(味酸微寒)、生姜三两(切,味辛温)、胶饴一升(味甘温)。

右六味,以水七升,煮取三升,去滓,内胶饴,更上微火,消解,温服一升,日三服。呕家不可用建中汤,以甜故也。

【今译】

伤寒证,患者阳脉滞涩,阴脉弦紧,应当有腹中拘急疼痛的症状,应先用小建中汤治疗。症状未解的,宜以小柴胡汤治疗。

Differentiation of pulse and syndrome / pattern [related to] taiyang disease and treatment (part 2)

【英译】

Line 100

Cold damage [disease], [characterized by] rough yang pulse, taut yin pulse and acute abdominal pain, [can be] treated first by Xiao Jianzhong Decoction (小建中汤, minor decoction for strengthening the middle). [If it is] not healed, Xiao Chaihu Decoction (小柴胡汤, minor bupleurum decoction) [can be] used.

Xiao Jianzhong Decoction (小建中汤, minor decoction for strengthening the middle) [is composed of] 3 *liang* of Guizhi (桂枝, cinnamon twig, Ramulus Cinnamomi) (bark-removed) pungent in taste and hot in property, 3 *liang* of Gancao (甘草, licorice, Radix Glycyrrhizae Praeparata) (broiled) sweet in taste and bland in property, 12 pieces of Dazao (大枣, jujube, Fructus Ziziphus Jujubae) (broken) sweet in taste and warm in property, 6 *liang* of Shaoyao (芍药, peony, Radix Paeoniae) sour in taste and slightly cold in property, 3 *liang* of Shengjiang (生姜, fresh ginger, Rhizoma Zingiberis Recens) cut, pungent in taste and warm in property and 1 *sheng* of Jiaoyi (胶饴, maltose, Maltosum) sweet in taste and warm in property.

These six ingredients are decocted in 7 *sheng* of water to get 3 *sheng* [after] boiling. [The decoction, after] removal of dregs, added with caramel and heated in mild fire to melt [caramel], is taken warm 1 *sheng* [each time] and three times a day. [Patient suffering from] vomiting cannot be treated by [Xiao] Jianzhong Decoction (小建中汤, minor decoction for strengthening the middle) because it is sweet.

【原文】

(一○一)

伤寒,中风,有柴胡证,但见一证便是,不必悉具。凡柴胡汤病证而下之,若柴胡证不罢者,复与柴胡汤,必蒸蒸而振,却复发热汗出而解。

【今译】

伤寒病中风后,有柴胡汤证的症候,只要见到一个证的就可确诊为柴胡汤证,不需要具备所有的症候。凡是柴胡汤证的都可用攻下法治疗,如果柴胡汤证没有解除,仍可以继续用柴胡汤进行治疗。患者服药后一定会高热战栗,然后发热汗出,使病得解。

【原文】

(一○二)

伤寒二三日,心中悸而烦者,小建中汤主之。

【今译】

伤寒病发作两三日,即出现心悸、烦闷现象,可用小建中汤治疗。

Differentiation of pulse and syndrome/pattern [related to] taiyang disease and treatment (part 2)

【英译】

Line 101

［In］ cold damage with wind stroke，［if］ there are [manifestations of] syndrome/pattern [to be treated by] Chaihu [Decoction (柴胡汤，bupleurum decoction)]，[even if] there is just one，[it still can be diagnosed as Chaihu Decoction (柴胡汤，bupleurum decoction) syndrome/pattern]. There is no need to find all [the necessary symptoms and signs]. [If] Chaihu Decoction (柴胡汤，bupleurum decoction) syndrome/pattern [is treated by] purgation but not eliminated，[it should be] treated by Chaihu Decoction (柴胡汤，bupleurum decoction). [After taking the decoction，the patient] will feel feverish and shivering. But high fever and perspiration will eliminate [the disease].

【英译】

Line 102

Cold damage [disease]，two or three days [after occurrence]，[characterized by] palpitation and dysphoria，[should be] treated by Xiao Jianzhong Decoction (小建中汤，minor decoction for strengthening the middle).

【原文】

(一〇三)

太阳病,过经十余日,反二三下之,后四五日,柴胡证仍在者,先与小柴胡汤;呕不止,心下急,郁郁微烦者,为未解也,与大柴胡汤下之则愈。

大柴胡汤方

柴胡半斤、黄芩三两、芍药三两、半夏半升(洗)、生姜五两(切)、枳实四枚(炙)、大枣十二枚(擘)。

右七味,以水一斗二升,煮取六升,去滓再煎,温服一升,日三服。一方加大黄二两,若不加,恐不为大柴胡汤也。

【今译】

太阳病,邪传少阳经十多天后,医生反而多次采用攻下法治疗。又经过四五天,如果柴胡证依然存在,可先用小柴胡汤治疗。如果出现呕吐不止,心下拘急,或者心中郁闷,略有烦躁的,是病情未解,用大柴胡汤攻下,即可痊愈。

Differentiation of pulse and syndrome / pattern [related to] taiyang disease and treatment (part 2)

【英译】

Line 103

Taiyang disease，after ten more days [of progress]，is repeatedly [treated by] purgation. After four or five days，Chaihu [Decoction (柴胡汤，bupleurum decoction)] syndrome/pattern still exists，Xiao Chaihu Decoction (小柴胡汤，minor bupleurum decoction) [can be used] to treat [it]. [If there are symptoms and signs of] repeated vomiting，abdominal contracture，depression and dysphoria，[it indicates that the disease is] not eliminated and Da Chaihu Decoction (大柴胡汤，major bupleurum decoction) [can be used] to heal [it].

Da Chaihu Decoction (大柴胡汤，major bupleurum decoction) [is composed of] 0.5 *jin* of Chaihu (柴胡，bupleurum，Radix Bupleuri)，3 *liang* of Huangqin (黄芩，scutellaria，Radix Scutellariae)，3 *liang* of Shaoyao (芍药，peony，Radix Paeoniae)，0.5 *sheng* of Banxia (半夏，pinellia，Rhizoma Pinelliae) washed，5 *liang* of Shengjiang (生姜，fresh ginger，Rhizoma Zingiberis Recens) (cut)，4 pieces of Zhishi (枳实，processed unripe bitter orange，Fructus Aurantii Immaturus) (broiled) and 12 pieces of Dazao (大枣，jujube，Fructus Ziziphus Jujubae) (broken).

These seven ingredients are decocted in 1 *dou* and 2 *sheng* of water to get 6 *sheng* [after] boiling. [The decoction，after] removal of dregs and being decocted again，is taken warm 1 *sheng* [each time] and three times a day. The other decoction must add 2 *liang* of Dahuang (大黄，rhubarb，Radix et Rhizoma Rhei)，otherwise [it] perhaps is not Da Chaihu Decoction (大柴胡汤，major bupleurum decoction).

【原文】

（一〇四）

伤寒十三日不解，胸胁满而呕，日晡所发潮热，已而微利。此本柴胡证，下之以不得利，今反利者，知医以丸药下之，此非其治也。潮热者，实也。先宜服小柴胡汤以解外，后以柴胡加芒硝汤主之。

柴胡加芒硝汤方

柴胡二两十六铢、黄芩一两、人参一两、甘草一两（炙）、生姜一两（切）、半夏二十铢（洗）、大枣四枚（擘）、芒硝二两。

右八味，以水四升，煮取两升，去滓，内芒硝更煮微沸，分温再服，不解更作。

【今译】

伤寒病，十三天后仍不解，胸胁满闷而呕吐，午后发潮热，并有轻微腹泻。这本来是大柴胡汤证，用攻下法治疗则不利。如今反而有利，说明医生用丸药攻下，此为错误治法。出现潮热的，是内有实邪之症，宜先服用小柴胡汤以解表邪，然后用柴胡加芒硝汤主治。

Differentiation of pulse and syndrome / pattern [related to] taiyang disease and treatment (part 2)

【英译】

Line 104

Cold damage [disease], not eliminated [after] thirteen days, [is characterized by] thoracic and costal fullness, vomiting, tidal fever in the late afternoon and slight diarrhea. It is originally Chaihu [Decoction] (柴胡汤, bupleurum decoction) syndrome/pattern and cannot be treated by purgation. [If the doctor], on the contrary, [treats it with] pills for purgation, it is a wrong treatment. Tidal fever [indicates] excess. [It] should be treated first by Xiao Chaihu Decoction (小柴胡汤, minor bupleurum decoction) in order to eliminate the external [pathogenic factors]. Afterwards Chaihu Decoction (柴胡汤, bupleurum decoction) added with Mangxiao (芒硝, mirabilite, Natrii Sulfas) [is used as] the main treatment.

Chaihu Decoction (柴胡汤, bupleurum decoction) added with Mangxiao (芒硝, mirabilite, Natrii Sulfas) [is composed of] 2 *liang* and 16 *zhu* of Chaihu (柴胡, bupleurum, Radix Buleuri), 1 *liang* of Huangqin (黄芩, scutellaria, Radix Scutellariae), 1 *liang* of Renshen (人参, ginseng, Radix Ginseng), 1 *liang* of Gancao (甘草, licorice, Radix Glycyrrhizae Praeparata) (broiled), 1 *liang* of Shengjiang (生姜, fresh ginger, Rhizoma Zingiberis Recens) (cut), 20 *zhu* of Banxia (半夏, pinellia, Rhizoma Pinelliae) (washed), 4 pieces of Dazao (大枣, jujube, Fructus Ziziphus Jujubae) (broken) and 2 *liang* of Mangxiao (芒硝, mirabilite, Natrii Sulfas).

These eight ingredients are decocted in 4 *sheng* of water to get 2 *sheng* [after] boiling. [After] removal of dregs, Mangxiao (芒硝, mirabilite, Natrii Sulfas) is put into [it] and boiled slightly. [The decoction is] divided [into two doses] and taken warm twice a day. [If there is] no elimination, [the decoction should be] taken again.

【原文】

(一○五)

伤寒十三日,过经谵语者,以有热也,当以汤下之。若小便利者,大便当鞭,而反下利,脉调和者,知医以丸药下之,非其治也。若自下利者,脉当微厥,今反和者,此为内实也,调胃承气汤主之。

【今译】

伤寒病发作十三日后,邪气入经而致谵语,此为有热的缘故,应当用攻下的汤药治疗。如果小便通利的,大便应当坚硬。如今反而发生下利,脉象且调和,说明是医生误用丸药攻下所致,属于错误治法。如果不是因误下而自动下利的,脉象应当微厥,现在脉象反而调和,这是内实的表现,宜用调胃承气汤治疗。

Differentiation of pulse and syndrome/pattern
[related to] taiyang disease and treatment (part 2)

【英译】

Line 105

[In] cold damage [disease], thirteen days [after occurrence], [there are] delirium and fever. [It] should [be treated] by decoction for purgation. If urination is normal, stool must be hard. But [there is] diarrhea [while] the pulse is in harmony, indicating [that] it is treated by pills for purgation, a wrong treatment. If there is diarrhea, the pulse should be slightly faint. [But] now [the pulse is] in harmony, indicating internal excess. [Therefore, it should be] treated by Tiaowei Chengqi Decoction (调胃承气汤, deccoction for regulating the stomach and harmonizing qi).

【原文】

（一〇六）

太阳病不解，热结膀胱，其人如狂，血自下，下者愈。其外不解者，尚未可攻，当先解其外。外解已，但少腹急结者，乃可攻之，宜桃核承气汤。

桃核承气汤方

桃仁五十个（去皮尖）、大黄四两、桂枝二两（去皮）、甘草二两（炙）、芒硝二两。

右五味，以水七升，煮取两升半，去滓，内芒硝，更上火微沸，下火，先食温服五合，日三服，当微利。

【今译】

太阳病未解，邪热内结于膀胱，患者出现有似发狂等症状。如果患者能自行下血，病就可痊愈。如果表症还未解除，就不能攻里，应当先解表。待解除后，只有少腹拘急的，才能攻里，宜用桃核承气汤方治疗。

Differentiation of pulse and syndrome/pattern [related to] taiyang disease and treatment (part 2)

【英译】

Line 106

Taiyang disease is not resolved and [pathogenic] heat acumulates in the bladder, [making] the patient appear manic. [If there is] spontaneous hemorrage, [the disease will] heal. [If] the external [syndrome/pattern] is not eliminated and [it is not the time] to purge the internal, the external [syndrome/pattern] should be relieved first. [If] the external [syndrome/pattern] is already eliminated but [there is still] lower abdominal spasm, [it] can [be treated by] Taohe Chengqi Decoction (桃核承气汤, peach kernel decoction for harmonizing qi) for purgation.

Taohe Chengqi Decoction (桃核承气汤, peach kernel decoction for harmonizing qi) [is composed of] 50 pieces of Taoren (桃仁, peach kernel, Semen Persicae) (peel-and-tips-removed), 4 *liang* of Dahuang (大黄, rhubarb, Radix et Rhizoma Rhei), 2 *liang* of Guizhi (桂枝, cinnamon twig, Ramulus Cinnamomi) (bark removed), 2 *liang* of Gancao (甘草, licorice, Radix Glycyrrhizae Praeparata) (broiled) and 2 *liang* of Mangxiao (芒硝, mirabilite, Natrii Sulfas).

These five ingredients are decocted in 7 *sheng* of water to get 2. 5 *sheng* [after] boiling. [After] dregs are removed, Mangxiao (芒硝, mirabilite, Natrii Sulfas) is put into [the decoction] and boiled again. [Before taking food], 5 *ge* [of decoction] is taken warm and three times a day. Mild diarrhea will occur [after taking the decoction].

【原文】

(一○七)

伤寒八九日,下之,胸满烦惊,小便不利,谵语,一身尽重,不可转侧者,柴胡加龙骨牡蛎汤主之。

柴胡加龙骨牡蛎汤方

柴胡四两,龙骨、黄芩、生姜(切)、铅丹、人参、桂枝(去皮)、茯苓各一两半,半夏二合半(洗),大黄二两,牡蛎一两半(熬),大枣六枚(擘)。

右十二味,以水八升,煮取四升,内大黄切如棋子,更煮一两沸,去滓,温服一升。本云柴胡汤,今加龙骨等。

【今译】

伤寒病,发作八九天后,误用攻下法,出现胸部满闷、烦躁惊惕、小便不畅、谵语、全身沉重、不能转侧的,宜用柴胡加龙骨牡蛎汤治疗。

【原文】

(一○八)

伤寒,腹满,谵语,寸口脉浮而紧,此肝乘脾也,名曰纵。刺期门。

【今译】

伤寒病,有腹部胀满、谵语、寸口脉浮而紧等症状,属肝木克伐脾土,所以名为"纵",可用针刺期门的方法治疗。

Differentiation of pulse and syndrome／pattern [related to] taiyang disease and treatment（part 2）

【英译】

Line 107

Eight to nine days [after occurrence of] cold damage [disease], purgation [used to treat it will cause] thoracic fullness, vexation, fear, delirium, heaviness of the body and difficulty to move. [It can be] treated by Chaihu Decoction（柴 胡 汤，bupleurum decoction）added with Longgu（龙骨，loong bone，Os Loong）and Muli（牡蛎，oyster shell，Concha Ostreae）.

Chaihu Decoction（柴胡汤，bupleurum decoction）added with Longgu（龙骨，loong bone，Os Loong）and Muli（牡蛎，oyster shell，Concha Ostreae）[is composed of] 4 *liang* of Chaihu（柴胡，bupleurum，Radix Bupleuri），1.5 *liang* of Longgu（龙骨，loong bone，Os Loong），1.5 *liang* of Huangqin（黄芩，scutellaria，Radix Scutellariae），1.5 *liang* of Shengjiang（生姜，fresh ginger，Rhizoma Zingiberis Recens）（cut），1.5 *liang* of Qiandan（铅丹，minium，Minium），1.5 *liang* of Renshen（人参，ginseng，Radix Ginseng），1.5 *liang* of Guizhi（桂枝，cinnamon twig，Ramulus Cinnamomi）（（bark removed）），1.5 *liang* of Fuling（茯苓，poria，Poria），2.5 *ge* of Banxia（半夏，pinellia，Rhizoma Pinelliae）（washed），2 *liang* of Dahuang（大黄，rhubarb，Radix et Rhizoma Rhei），1.5 *liang* of Muli（牡蛎，oyster shell，Concha Ostreae）（simmer）and 6 pieces of Dazao（大枣，jujube，Fructus Ziziphus Jujubae）（broken）.

These 12 ingredients are decocted in 8 *sheng* of water to get 4 *sheng* [after] boiling. [Then] Dahuang（大黄，rhubarb，Radix et Rhizoma Rhei）is [cut into small pieces,] put into [the decoction] and boiled again for once or twice. [Afterwards,] the dregs are removed [and the decoction] is taken 1 *sheng* warm [each time]. The old edition says that Chaihu Decoction（柴胡汤，bupleurum decoction）can be added with Longgu（龙骨，loong bone，Os Loong）[and other ingredients].

【原文】

(一〇九)

伤寒发热,啬啬恶寒,大渴欲饮水,其腹必满,自汗出,小便利,其病欲解,此肝乘肺也,名曰横。刺期门。

【今译】

伤寒病,病人有发热、啬啬恶寒、口感大渴而想喝水症状的,必定会有腹满。如果自汗出,小便通利,病就将解除。这属于肝克肺,叫做"横",可以针刺期门的方法治疗。

【原文】

(一一〇)

太阳病二日,反躁,凡熨其背而大汗出,大热入胃,胃中水竭,躁烦,必发谵语,十余日,振栗,自下利者,此为欲解也。故其汗从腰以下不得汗,欲小便不得,反呕,欲失溲,足下恶风,大便鞕,小便当数,而反不数及不多,大便已,头卓然而痛,其人足心必热,谷气下流故也。

【今译】

太阳病发作的第二天,患者出现烦躁不安的症状,医生反而用热熨患者的背部,导致大热之邪乘虚内入于胃,使胃中津液枯竭,出现躁扰不宁、谵语等病症。十多天后,若患者出现全身颤抖、腹泻的,说明疾

Differentiation of pulse and syndrome/pattern
[related to] taiyang disease and treatment (part 2)

【英译】

Line 108

Cold damage, [characterized by] abdominal fullness, delirium, floating and tight pulse in the Cunkou region, [is caused by] the liver invading the spleen, known as Zong (vertical invasion). [It can be treated by] needling Qimen (LR14).

【英译】

Line 109

Cold damage, [characterized by] fever, chillness, aversion to cold, great thirst with desire to drink water, abdominal fullness, spontaneous sweating and normal urination with desire to eliminate the disease, [is caused by] the liver invading the lung, known as Heng (transverse invasion) [and can be treated by] needling Qimen (LR 14).

【英译】

Line 110

[In] the second day of taiyang disease, [the patient begins to suffer from] vexation. [If the doctor] scorches his back, [it will cause] profuse sweating, invasion of excessive heat into the stomach, exhaustion of fluid in the stomach, vexation and delirium. [After] ten more days [of treatment and progress, if there are] shivering and diarrhea, [the disease is] about to heal. [There may

病即将解除。如果采用火攻法治疗,病人腰以下部位将不出汗,反见呕吐,足底下感觉冰凉,大便干硬,本应当小便频数,但反而不频数而量少,解大便后头部猛然疼痛,并且脚心发热,这是谷气向下流的缘故。

【原文】

(———)

太阳病中风,以火劫发汗。邪风被火热,血气流溢,失其常度。两阳相熏灼,其身发黄。阳盛则欲衄,阴虚小便难。阴阳俱虚竭,身体则枯燥,但头汗出,剂颈而还,腹满,微喘,口干咽烂,或不大便。久则谵语,甚者至哕,手足躁扰,捻衣摸床,小便利者,其人可治。

【今译】

太阳病中风后,如果用火法强制发汗,风邪被火热所迫,血气失去正常规律而流溢,风与火相互熏灼,使病人身体发黄,阳热亢盛就会出现衄血,阴液亏虚就会使小便短少。气血俱虚就会出现身体枯燥,仅头部出汗,到颈部为止,腹部胀满,微微气喘,口干咽喉溃烂,或者大便不通,时间久了就会出现谵语,严重的则会有呃逆、手足躁扰、捻衣摸床等症。如果小便通畅,患者尚可救治。

Differentiation of pulse and syndrome / pattern [related to] taiyang disease and treatment (part 2)

also appear such symptoms and signs of] no perspiration below the waist, difficulty in urination, vomiting, incontinence of urine, aversion to wind at the feet, hard stool, urination that should be frequent and profuse but infrequent and little, headache after defecation and feverish soles. [This is due to] downward flow of cereal qi.

【英译】

Line 111

[To treat] wind stroke in taiyang disease, scorching therapy [can be used to] induce perspiration. Heated by fire, pathogenic wind [will cause] abnormal flow of blood and qi, fumigation and scorching of both yang (wind and fire) and yellow skin. [If] yang is exuberant, [it will cause] epistaxis; [if] yin is deficient, [it will cause] dysuria. [If] both yin and yang (qi and blood) are deficient or exhausted, [it will cause] dryness of the body, perspiration over the head to the neck, abdominal fullness, slight panting, dryness of the mouth, ulceration of the throat, or constipation. [If] continuing for a long time, [it will cause] delirium, or even nausea, restless movement of hands and feet, carphology and normal urination. Such a patient is still curable.

【原文】

(一一二)

伤寒,脉浮,医以火迫劫之,亡阳,必惊狂,卧起不安者,桂枝去芍药加蜀漆牡蛎龙骨救逆汤主之。

桂枝去芍药加蜀漆牡蛎龙骨救逆汤方

桂枝三两(去皮)、甘草二两(炙)、生姜三两(切)、大枣十二枚(擘)、牡蛎五两(熬)、蜀漆三两(洗去腥)、龙骨四两。

右七味,以水一斗二升,先煮蜀漆,减二升,内诸药,煮取三升,去滓,温服一升。本云桂枝汤,今去芍药加蜀漆牡蛎龙骨。

【今译】

伤寒病,脉象浮,本应当发汗解表,医生反而用火治法强行发汗,导致阳亡,患者出现惊恐狂乱、坐卧不安等症状,宜用桂枝去芍药加蜀漆牡蛎龙骨救逆汤主治。

Differentiation of pulse and syndrome / pattern
[related to] taiyang disease and treatment (part 2)

【英译】

Line 112

[If syndrome/pattern of] cold damage with floating pulse is treated by scorching [therapy for inducing perspiration, it will cause] loss of yang, fright, mania and restlessness in sitting and lying. [It should be] treated by Guizhi Decoction (桂枝汤, cinnamon twig decoction) with Shaoyao (芍药, penoy, Radix Paseoniae) removed and Shuqi (蜀漆, dichroa, Dichroa febrifuga Lour), Longgu (龙骨, loong bone, Os Loong) and Muli (牡蛎, oyster shell, Concha Ostreae) added.

Guizhi Decoction (桂枝汤, cinnamon twig decoction) with Shaoyao (芍药, penoy, Radix Paseoniae) removed and Shuqi (蜀漆, dichroa, Dichroa febrifuga Lour), Longgu (龙骨, loong bone, Os Loong) and Muli (牡蛎, oyster shell, Concha Ostreae) added [is composed of] 3 *liang* of Guizhi (桂枝, cinnamon twig, Ramulus Cinnamomi) (bark-removed), 2 *liang* of Gancao (甘草, licorice, Radix Glycyrrhizae Praeparata) (broiled), 3 *liang* of Shengjiang (生姜, fresh ginger, Rhizoma Ziziphi Jujubae) (cut), 12 pieces of Dazao (大枣, jujube, Fructus Ziziphus Jujubae) (broken), 5 *liang* of Muli (牡蛎, oyster shell, Concha Ostreae) (simmer), 3 *liang* of Shuqi (蜀漆, dichora, Dichroa febrifuga Lour) (washed to remove fish smell) and 4 *liang* of Longgu (龙骨, loong bone, Os Loong).

These seven ingredients are decocted in 1 *dou* and 2 *sheng* of water. Shuqi (蜀漆, dichroa, Dichroa febrifuga Lour) is decocted first to reduce 2 *sheng* of water. [Then] the other ingredients are put into it and decocted to get 3 *sheng* [after] boiling. [After] removal of dregs, [the decoction] is taken warm 1 *sheng* [each time]. The old edition says that in Guizhi Decoction (桂枝汤, cinnamon twig decoction), Shaoyao (芍药, peony, Radix Paseoniae) is removed, Shuqi (蜀漆, dichroa, Dichroa febrifuga Lour), Longgu (龙骨, loong bone, Os Loong) and Muli (牡蛎, oyster shell, Concha Ostreae) are added.

【原文】

(一一三)

形作伤寒,其脉不弦紧而弱,弱者必渴,被火必谵语,弱者发热,脉浮,解之当汗出愈。

【今译】

疾病的表现类似太阳伤寒证,但其脉搏却不弦紧反而弱,脉弱必然出现口渴现象。若误用火攻,必然出现谵语等病症。初起脉弱的,将发热,脉将浮,解表则汗出,汗出则疾病可愈。

【原文】

(一一四)

太阳病,以火熏之,不得汗,其人必躁。到经不解,必清血,名为火邪。

【今译】

太阳病,用火熏法治疗后,如果没有汗出,患者必然发生烦躁。如邪入经而未解,必然会发生便血,所以名为火邪。

Differentiation of pulse and syndrome/pattern [related to] taiyang disease and treatment (part 2)

【英译】

Line 113

[The disease is] similar to cold damage [disease in manifestations], [however] the pulse is not taut and tight, but weak. [If the pulse is] weak, [the patient is] certainly thirsty. [If treated by] purgation with fire, [the patient will become] delirious. [At the early stage of this disease, there are symptoms and signs of] weak pulse and fever, diaphoresis [can be used] to eliminate it.

【英译】

Line 114

[To treat] taiyang disease, fire fumigation is unable to induce sweating but causes vexation. [When it has already] transmitted to [the related] meridians but still is not eliminated, [it will] inevitably lead to bloody stool, known as pathogenic fire.

【原文】

(一一五)

脉浮，热甚，而反灸之，此为实。实以虚治，因火而动，必咽燥，吐血。

【今译】

脉象浮，发热甚，却反用温灸法治疗，此为实证。如果把实证当做虚证治疗，会使火邪内攻，必然会出现咽喉干燥、吐血等症状。

【原文】

(一一六)

微数之脉，慎不可灸，因火为邪，则为烦逆，追虚逐实，血散脉中，火气虽微，内攻有力，焦骨伤筋，血难复也。脉浮，宜以汗解。用火灸之，邪无从出，因火而盛，病从腰以下必重而痹，名火逆也。欲自解者，必当先烦，烦乃有汗而解。何以知之？脉浮，故知汗出解。

【今译】

患者脉象微数，治疗时不可用灸法。如果误用温灸，就会使其成为火邪，引起烦乱不安的症状出现。阴血本虚反用灸法，使阴更伤；热本属实，用火法更使内热增强，会使血液流散于脉中，使其运行失常。灸火虽然微弱，但内攻却有力，损伤筋骨，使血液难以恢复正常。脉象浮，

Differentiation of pulse and syndrome / pattern [related to] taiyang disease and treatment (part 2)

【英译】

Line 115

[If the disease with] floating pulse and severe fever is treated by moxibustion, [it is a wrong treatment, for] this is an excess [syndrome/pattern]. To treat excess as deficiency will cause dryness of the throat and blood vomiting due to fire [stimulation].

【英译】

Line 116

[If the patient's] pulse is slightly rapid, moxibustion cannot be used. [Wrong use of moxibustion will make] fire pathogenic, causing vexation, worsening deficiency and excess and driving the blood to flow abnormally in the vessels. [Though] fire [from moxibustion] is not strong, [it] can strongly attack the internal, scorching the bones, injuring the sinews and making it difficult to smooth [the circulation of] the blood. Floating pulse can be relieved by diaphoresis. [If] moxibustion is used, pathogenic factors cannot be eliminated [through diaphoresis]. [On the contrary, pathogenic heat will become] exuberant due to moxibustion, [resulting in] heaviness and numbness below the waist, known as adverse fire. [When the disease] is about to heal, there must be vexation first, [followed by] sweating and elimination. How to understand such a procedure? [The reason is that] floating pulse indicates sweating [and sweating is helpful for]

治疗时宜用发汗解表法。如果用灸法治疗，表邪就不能通过发汗解除，反而因火法而炽盛，使得从腰以下沉重而麻痹，这就叫火逆。如果病将自行痊愈的，患者一定会先出现心烦不安，但心烦而有汗出的，病必愈解。怎么知道的呢？因为脉浮，故而得知汗出而病解。

【原文】

(一一七)

烧针令其汗，针处被寒，核起而赤者，必发奔豚，气从少腹上冲心者，灸其核上各一壮，与桂枝加桂汤，更加桂枝二两也。

桂枝加桂汤方

桂枝五两(去皮)、芍药三两、生姜三两(切)、甘草二两(炙)、大枣十二枚(擘)。

右五味，以水七升，煮取三升，去滓，温服一升。本云桂枝汤，今加桂满五两，所以加桂者，以能泄奔豚气也。

【今译】

用烧针法发汗，针刺部位受到寒邪侵袭，就会出现红色核块，必然引发奔豚。如果气从少腹上冲心胸的，可用艾火在其核上各灸一壮，内服桂枝加桂汤，即桂枝汤原方再加桂枝二两。

Differentiation of pulse and syndrome / pattern
[related to] taiyang disease and treatment (part 2)

eliminating [the disease].

【英译】

Line 117

To induce sweating [by acupuncture with] heated needle [will result in] coldness in the needled region and red nodule, consequently causing running piglet and qi rushing from the lower abdomen to the heart. [Externally] moxibustion [can be used to fumigate] the nodule with one cone [of moxia]. [Internally] Guizhi Decoction (桂枝汤, cinnamon twig decoction) added with 2 *liang* of Guizhi (桂枝, cinnamon twig, Ramulus Cinnamomi) [can be used].

Guizhi Decoction (桂枝汤, cinnamon twig decoction) added with 2 *liang* of Guizhi (桂枝, cinnamon twig, Ramulus Cinnamomi) [is composed of] 5 *liang* of Guizhi (桂枝, cinnamon twig, Ramulus Cinnamomi) (bark removed), 3 *liang* of Shaoyao (芍药, peony, Radix Paeoniae), 3 *liang* of Shengjiang (生姜, fresh ginger, Rhizoma Zingiberis Recens) (cut), 2 *liang* of Gancao (甘草, licorice, Radix Glycyrrhizae Praeparata) (broiled) and 12 pieces of Dazao (大枣, jujube, Fructus Ziziphus Jujubae) (broken).

These five ingredients are decocted in 7 *sheng* of water to get 3 *sheng* [after] boiling. The dregs are removed and [the decoction is] taken warm 1 *sheng* [each time]. The old edition says that [it is necessary] to increase Guizhi (桂枝, cinnamon twig, Ramulus Cinnamomi) into 5 *liang* in order to eliminate qi of running piglet.

【原文】

(一一八)

火逆下之，因烧针，烦躁者，桂枝甘草龙骨牡蛎汤主之。

桂枝甘草龙骨牡蛎汤

桂枝一两(去皮)、甘草二两(炙)、牡蛎二两(熬)、龙骨二两。

右四味，以水五升，煮取二升半，去滓，温服八合，日三服。

【今译】

火攻之后又用火针攻下，必然出现烦躁不安等症状，宜用桂枝甘草龙骨牡蛎汤治疗。

【原文】

(一一九)

太阳伤寒者，加温针必惊也。

【今译】

太阳伤寒病，使用温针治疗，必然引起惊栗。

Differentiation of pulse and syndrome / pattern [related to] taiyang disease and treatment (part 2)

【英译】

Line 118

[Application of] scorching therapy [followed by] purgation will cause vexation due to [acupuncture with] heated needle. [It can be] treated by Guizhi Gancao Longgu Muli Decoction (桂枝甘草龙骨牡蛎汤, cinnamon twig, licorice, loong bone and oyster shell decoction).

Guizhi Gancao Longgu Muli Decoction (桂枝甘草龙骨牡蛎汤, cinnamon twig, licorice, loong bone and oyster shell decoction) [is composed of] 1 *liang* of Guizhi (桂枝, cinnamon twig, Ramulus Cinnamomi) (bark removed), 2 *liang* of Gancao (甘草, licorice, Radix Glycyrrhizae Praeparata) (broiled), 2 *liang* of Muli (牡蛎, oyster shell, Concha Ostreae) (simmer) and 2 *liang* of Longgu (龙骨, loong bone, Os Loong).

These four ingredients are decocted in 5 *sheng* of water to get 2.5 *sheng* [after] boiling. The dregs are removed and [the decoction is] taken warm 8 *ge* [each time] and three times a day.

【英译】

Line 119

[If] taiyang cold damage [disease is treated by acupuncture with] warm needle, [it will cause] tremble.

【原文】

(一二〇)

太阳病,当恶寒、发热,今自汗出,反不恶寒、发热,关上脉细数者,以医吐之过也。一二日吐之者,腹中饥,口不能食;三四日吐之者,不喜糜粥,欲食冷食,朝食暮吐,以医吐之所致也,此为小逆。

【今译】

太阳病,应当有恶寒、发热等症状。如今患者自汗出,反而不恶寒、不发热,关脉细数,这是医生误用吐法治疗的缘故。病发一二日后用吐法治疗,患者将出现腹中饥、口不能食等症状。病发三四日后用吐法治疗,患者不喜食用糜粥,想用餐时则食用冷餐,出现朝食暮吐等症状,这就是医生误用吐法治疗所致,这就叫小逆。

【原文】

(一二一)

太阳病,吐之,但太阳病当恶寒,今反不恶寒,不欲近衣,此为吐之内烦也。

【今译】

太阳病,用吐法治疗。但太阳病患者应当恶寒,如今反而不恶寒,也不想多穿衣,这就是误用吐法而引起的心中烦躁所致。

Differentiation of pulse and syndrome/pattern [related to] taiyang disease and treatment (part 2)

【英译】

Line 120

[In] taiyang disease, [there should be] aversion to cold and fever. [But] now [there are] spontaneous sweating, no aversion to cold, no fever, and thin and rapid pulse due to wrong use of vomiting therapy. [To treat the disease with] vomiting [therapy] one or two days [after occurrence will make the patient feel] hungry but difficult to eat. [To treat the disease with] vomiting [therapy] three or four days [after occurrence will make the patient] unwilling to take porridge, but desire to take cold food. [The patient will] vomit in the evening what he has taken in the morning due to [wrong use of] vomiting [treatment]. [That is why] it is called minor adverseness.

【英译】

Line 121

[In] taiyang disease originally [there is] aversion to cold, but [when treated by] vomiting [therapy], there is no aversion to cold and [the patient] does not want to wear clothes. This is internal dysphoria [due to wrong use of] vomiting [therapy].

【原文】

(一二二)

病人脉数,数为热,当消谷引食,而反吐者,此以发汗,令阳气微,膈气虚,脉乃数也。数为客热,不能消谷,以胃中虚冷,故吐也。

【今译】

病人脉数,脉数为热象,会加快消化食物,增加胃口。如今反而呕吐,这是因为使用发汗法,使得阳气微弱,膈间正气虚弱,这就是导致脉象频数的原因。这种频数的脉象是邪热的表现,不能加快食物消化,因为胃中有虚冷,所以才引起呕吐。

【原文】

(一二三)

太阳病,过经十余日,心下温温欲吐,而胸中痛,大便反溏,腹微满,郁郁微烦,先此时自极吐下者,与调胃承气汤。若不尔者,不可与。但欲呕,胸中痛,微溏者,此非柴胡汤证,以呕故知极吐下也。

【今译】

太阳病,经过十余天的发展,患者心下温温欲吐,胸中疼痛,大便反而溏稀,腹部微有胀满,心中郁郁微烦,此为吐下法所致,可用调胃承气汤治疗。如果不属于这种情况,就不可用此法治疗。如果患者想呕吐,胸中疼痛,大便略微溏稀,这不是柴胡汤证,因患者想呕吐,所以可以推知是大吐大下所致。

Differentiation of pulse and syndrome / pattern [related to] taiyang disease and treatment（part 2）

【英译】

Line 122

The patient's pulse is rapid. Rapid [pulse] indicates [pathogenic] heat [that promotes] digestion [and increases] appetite. But now there is vomiting. This is due to [wrong use of] diaphoresis，leading to declination of yang qi and deficiency of qi in the diaphragm. [That is why] the pulse is rapid. [Such] rapid [pulse is a manifestation of] false heat [that in fact] cannot digest food because [there is] deficiency-cold in the stomach. That is why [there is] vomiting.

【英译】

Line 123

Taiyang disease，after ten more days [progress]，[there are symptoms and signs of] vexation with desire to vomit，chest pain，sloppy stool，slightly abdominal fullness，depression and certain restlessness. [If caused by] vomiting [therapy] or purgation，[it can be treated by] Tiaowei Chengqi Decoction（调胃承气汤，decoction for regulating the stomach and harmonizing qi）. If [it is] not such a case，[it] should not [be treated in such a way]. [If there are symptoms and signs of] desire to vomit，chest pain and slightly sloppy stool，but not [belonging to] Chaihu Decoction（柴胡汤，bupleurum decoction） syndrome/pattern，[it is caused by] severe vomiting and purgation.

【原文】

(一二四)

太阳病,六七日表证仍在,脉微而沉,反不结胸,其人发狂者,以热在下焦,少腹当鞕满,小便自利者,下血乃愈。所以然者,以太阳随经,瘀热在里故也。抵当汤主之。

抵当汤方

水蛭(熬)、虻虫各三十个(去翅足,熬)、桃仁二十个(去皮尖)、大黄三两(酒洗)。

右四味,以水五升,煮取三升,去滓,温服一升,不下更服。

【今译】

太阳病,发作六七日后表证仍在,脉象微而沉,但反而无结胸之相。如果患者有发狂之相,是因为热在下焦,使少腹硬结闷满,小便自利。通过下血则可使病愈。之所以如此,是因为病邪从太阳经入内,使得内有瘀热的缘故。宜用抵当汤主治。

【原文】

(一二五)

太阳病身黄,脉沉结,少腹鞕,小便不利者,为无血也。小便自利,其人如狂者,血证谛也。抵当汤主之。

Differentiation of pulse and syndrome / pattern [related to] taiyang disease and treatment（part 2）

【英译】

Line 124

Taiyang disease，still remaining after six or seven days，[is characterized by] faint and sunken pulse and absence of chest bind. [If] the patient is manic，[it is due to] heat in the lower energizer，hardness and fullness of the lower abdomen and spontaneous urination. [It can be] cured by resolving blood stasis. The reason why this [is so is that the pathogenic factors in] taiyang [transmit into the internal] along [certain] meridians，[consequently leading to binding of blood] stasis and [pathogenic] heat in the internal. [Therefore it should be] treated by Didang Decoction（抵当汤，decoction for prevention）.

Didang Decoction（抵当汤，decoction for prevention）[is composed of] 30 pieces of Shuizhi（水蛭，leech，Hirudo）simmered，30 pieces of Mengchong（虻虫，tabanus，Tabanus）simmered with wings and legs removed，20 pieces of Taoren（桃仁，peach kernel，Semen Persicae）peel and tips removed and 3 *liang* of Dahuang（大黄，rhubarb，Radix et Rhizoma Rhei）washed it with liquor.

These four ingredients are decocted in 5 *sheng* of water to 3 *sheng* [after] boiling. The dregs are removed and [the decoction is] taken warm 1 *sheng* [each time]. [If blood stasis is] not resolved，[the decoction should be] taken again.

【英译】

Line 125

Taiyang disease [is characterized by] yellow skin，sunken and

【今译】

太阳病,出现身体发黄,脉象沉结,小腹坚硬的症状。如果小便不通畅,并非蓄血症。如果小便通畅,但患者有狂乱征兆的,属蓄血发黄证,宜用抵当汤主治。

【原文】

(一二六)

伤寒有热,少腹满,应小便不利,今反利者,为有血也,当下之,不可余药,宜抵当丸。

抵当丸方

水蛭二十个(熬)、虻虫二十五个(去翅足,熬)、桃仁十五个(去皮尖)、大黄三两。

右四味,捣分四丸,以水一升,煮一丸,取七合服之。晬时当下血,若不下者,更服。

【今译】

伤寒病,身上有热,少腹胀满,应当有小便不利之症,但现在小便反而通利,为下焦蓄血的征象,治当以祛除瘀血为主,不是其他药能有效治疗,宜用抵当丸主治。

Differentiation of pulse and syndrome/pattern [related to] taiyang disease and treatment（part 2）

bound pulse，hardness in the lower abdomen and dysuria，[it is] not blood [amassment]．[If] urination is normal [but] the patient is manic，[it is] a blood [stasis] syndrome/pattern [and should be] treated by Didang Decoction（抵当汤，decoction for prevention）．

【英译】

Line 126

[In] cold damage with heat and lower abdominal fullness，there should be dysuria．[But] now there is normal urination because there is blood [stasis in the lower energizer]，[and therefore] should [be treated by] purgation．Other medicinals cannot be used，only Didang Pill（抵当丸，pill for prevention）is appropriate．

Didang Pill（抵当丸，pill for prevention）[is composed of] 20 pieces of Shuizhi（水蛭，leech，Hirudo）simmered，25 pieces of Mengchong（虻虫，tabanus，Tabanus）simmered with wings and legs removed，15 pieces of Taoren（桃仁，peach kerneal，Semen Persicae）（peel and tips removed）and 3 *liang* of Dahuang（大黄，rhubarb，Radix et Rhizoma Rhei）．

These four ingredients are divided into four pills and decocted in 1 *sheng* of water to boil one pill and get 7 *ge*．[The decoction] is taken [together with the dregs]．[If blood stasis is] not resolved，[the decoction should be] taken again．

【原文】

(一二七)

太阳病,小便利者,以饮水多,必心下悸;小便少者,必苦里急也。

【今译】

太阳病,小便畅利的,是因为饮水过多所致,必然会有心悸之症。如果小便短少不畅,必然出现小腹部胀满急迫不舒的症状。

Differentiation of pulse and syndrome/pattern
[related to] taiyang disease and treatment (part 2)

【英译】

Line 127

[In] taiyang disease, smooth urination is due to drinking copious water [and will] certainly cause palpitation. [If] urine is scanty, [there will appear lower abdominal] fullness and urgency.

辨太阳病脉证并治下

【原文】

(一二八)

问曰：病有结胸，有脏结，其状何如？答曰：按之痛，寸脉浮，关脉沉，名曰结胸也。

【今译】

问：病症有胸结，有脏结，其表现会是什么样的呢？

答：胸脘部按则疼痛，寸部脉浮，关部脉沉，即为"结胸"的表现。

【原文】

(一二九)

何谓脏结？答曰：如结胸状，饮食如故，时时下利，寸脉浮，关脉小细沉紧，名曰脏结。舌上白胎滑者，难治。

【今译】

问：什么叫脏结症？

答：与结胸的症状相似，但饮食如常，时时腹泻，寸部脉浮，关部脉小细而沉紧，这就叫做脏结症。舌苔白而滑腻的，很难治疗。

Differentiation of pulse and syndrome/pattern [related to] taiyang disease and treatment (part 3)

【英译】

Line 128

Question: What are the manifestations of the disease [characterized by] chest bind and visceral bind?

Answer: [If the chest is] painful under pressure, the cun pulse is floating and guan pulse is sunken, [it is] called chest bind.

【英译】

Line 129

[Question]: What is visceral bind?

Answer: [It is] similar to the manifestations of chest bind [with the symptoms and signs of] normal appetite, frequent diarrhea, floating cun pulse, and thin, sunken and tight guan pulse. [It is thus] called visceral bind. [If] the tongue fur is white and slippery, [it is] difficult to treat.

【原文】

(一三〇)

脏结无阳证,不往来寒热,其人反静,舌上胎滑者,不可攻也。

【今译】

脏结没有阳性的见证,无寒热往来,患者反而安静,舌上胎滑的,不可用攻下法治疗。

【原文】

(一三一)

病发于阳,而反下之,热入因作结胸;病发于阴,而反下之,因作痞也。所以成结胸者,以下之太早故也。结胸者,项亦强,如柔痉状,下之则和,宜大陷胸丸。

大陷胸丸方

大黄半斤、葶苈子半升(熬)、芒硝半升、杏仁半升(去皮尖熬黑)。

右四味,捣筛二味,内杏仁、芒硝,合研如脂,和散,取如弹丸一枚,别捣甘遂末一钱匕,白蜜二合,水两升,煮取一升,温顿服之,一宿乃下,如不下,更服,取下为效,禁如药法。

【今译】

太阳病,邪气盛实,误用下法,邪热内陷,就会成为结胸。发病于里,正气不足,误用下法,就会成为痞证。所以成为结胸,是因为攻下太早的缘故。结胸证,项部也会强直,如同柔痉一样,以攻下治疗,强直就可转为柔和,可用大陷胸丸。

Differentiation of pulse and syndrome/pattern [related to] taiyang disease and treatment (part 3)

【英译】

Line 130

[In] visceral bind, [if] there are no yang [heat] syndrome/pattern and alternate chillness and heat, [but] the tongue fur is slippery, [it] cannot [be treated by] purgation.

【英译】

Line 131

[If] the disease originating from yang [is treated by] purgation, [pathogenic] heat will enter the internal and cause chest bind. [If] the disease originating from yin [is treated by] purgation, [it will] cause stagnancy. Thus chest bind results from early purgation. [In] chest bind, the neck is also stiff like mild tetany. [If treated by] purgation, [it will become] soft. [This pill] should be treated by Da Xianxiong Pill (大陷胸丸,major pill for resolving chest sinking).

Da Xianxiong Pill (大陷胸丸,major pill for resolving chest sinking) [is composed of] 0.5 *jin* of Dahuang (大黄, rhubarb, Radx et Rhizoma Rhei), 0.5 *sheng* of Tinglizi (葶苈子, semen tingli, Semen Lepidii Descurainiae) (simmered), 0.5 *sheng* of Mangxiao (芒硝, mirabilite, Natrii Sulfas) and 0.5 *sheng* of Xingren (杏仁, apricot kernel, Semen Armeniacae Amarum) (peel and tips removed, simmered to be black).

Among these four ingredients, Dahuang (大黄, rhubarb, Radx et Rhizoma Rhei) and Tinglizi (葶苈子, semen tingli, Semen Lepidii Descurainiae) are pounded, Mangxiao (芒硝, mirabilite, Natrii Sulfas) and Xingren (杏仁, apricot kernel, Semen Armeniacae Amarum) are ground. [These four pounded and ground ingredients] are mixed like fat [and the pills are made as big] as bullets. One spoonful of Gansui (甘遂, kansui, Radix Euphorbiae Kansui) is pounded [into powder with] 2 *ge* of Baimi (白蜜, honey, Mel) in 2 *sheng* of water. [It is] decocted to get 1 *sheng* [after] boiling. [The decoction is] taken warm [and the disease will be] resolved overnight. If it is not eliminated, [the decoction should be] taken again till [there is] effectiveness. These instructions must be followed.

【原文】

(一三二)

结胸证,其脉浮大者,不可下,下之则死。

【今译】

结胸症,其脉象浮大,治疗不能用攻下法,若攻下则会导致病人死亡。

【原文】

(一三三)

结胸证悉具,烦躁者亦死。

【今译】

结胸症,临床症候全部具备,患者烦躁不宁的,也是死候。

Differentiation of pulse and syndrome / pattern [related to] taiyang disease and treatment (part 3)

【英译】

Line 132

Chest bind syndrome/pattern with floating and large pulse cannot [be treated by] purgation. [If] purgation is used, [it will lead to] death.

【英译】

Line 133

[If] all [the concerned symptoms and signs are observed] in chest bind syndrome/pattern and [the patient feels] restless and dysphoric, [it is] fatal.

【原文】

（一三四）

太阳病，脉浮而动数，浮则为风，数则为热，动则为痛，数则为虚。头痛，发热，微盗汗出，而反恶寒者，表未解也。医反下之，动数变迟，膈内拒痛，胃中空虚，客气动膈，短气躁烦，心中懊憹，阳气内陷，心下因鞕，则为结胸。大陷胸汤主之。若不结胸，但头汗出，余处无汗，剂颈而还，小便不利，身必发黄。

大陷胸汤方

大黄六两（去皮）、芒硝一升、甘遂一钱匕。

右三味，以水六升，先煮大黄，取二升，去滓，内芒硝，煮一两沸，内甘遂末，温服一升，得快利，止后服。

【今译】

太阳病，脉象浮而动数，脉象浮为风邪在表，脉象数为体中有热，脉象动则为痛，脉象数则为虚。头痛，发热，轻微盗汗，反而恶寒等症状，说明太阳表症未除。医生反而用攻下法治疗，导致动数脉变为迟脉，胸胁疼痛拒按，胃中空虚，短气，烦躁不安，心中懊憹，阳气内陷，心下硬结，这样结胸症就出现了。主治用大陷胸汤。如果没有形成结胸，只有头部汗出，到颈部为止，其他部位没有汗出，小便不畅，则身体发黄，为湿热郁蒸发黄症。

Differentiation of pulse and syndrome / pattern [related to] taiyang disease and treatment (part 3)

【英译】

Line 134

[In] taiyang disease, the pulse is floating, moving and rapid. Floating [pulse] indicates [invasion of pathogenic] wind [into superficies], rapid [pulse] indicates heat, moving [pulse] indicates pain and rapid [pulse] also indicates deficiency. [If there are symptoms and signs of] headache, fever, light sweating and aversion to cold, [it indicates that] external [syndrome/pattern] is not relieved. [If treated by] purgation, [it will result in] moving and rapid pulse changing into slow [pulse], severe pain in the diaphragm, emptiness and deficiency of the stomach, [pathogenic] qi attacking the diaphragm, shortness of breath, dysphoria, vexation, internal sinking of yang qi and lump below the heart. This is chest bind and [should be] treated by Da Xianxiong Decoction (大陷胸汤, major decoction for resolving chest sinking). If no chest bind [is formed] and [there are just] sweating over the head to the neck and dysuria, the skin must be yellow.

Da Xianxiong Decoction (大陷胸汤, major decoction for resolving chest sinking) [is composed of] 6 *liang* of Dahuang (大黄, rhubarb, Radix et Rhizoma Rhei) (bark removed), 1 *sheng* of Mangxiao (芒硝, mirabilite, Natrii Sulfas) and 1 *qianbi* (about 1 gram) of Gansui (甘遂, kansui root, Radix Euphorbiae Kansui).

These three ingredients are decocted in 6 *sheng* of water. Dahuang (大黄, rhubarb, Radix et Rhizoma Rhei) is decocted first to get 2 *sheng* of water [after] boiling. The dregs are removed and Mangxiao (芒硝, mirabilite, Natrii Sulfas) is put into it and boiled once or twice. [Then] Gansui (甘遂, kansui root, Radix Euphorbiae Kansui) powder is put into it. [The decoction] is taken warm 1 *sheng* [each time]. [When] there is sloppy stool, cease taking [the decoction].

【原文】

（一三五）

伤寒六七日，结胸热实，脉沉而紧，心下痛，按之石鞭者，大陷胸汤主之。

【今译】

伤寒病发作六七天后，出现热实结胸，脉象沉而紧，心下疼痛，按之像石头一样坚硬，宜用大陷胸汤主治。

【原文】

（一三六）

伤寒十余日，热结在里，复往来寒热者，与大柴胡汤；但结胸，无大热者，此为水结在胸胁也。但头微汗出者，大陷胸汤主之。

【今译】

伤寒病发作十多日，热邪结于里，又有往来寒热，可用大柴胡汤治疗。如果只有结胸症状，也无大热，这是因水结于胸胁的缘故。如果仅头部微微汗出，宜用大陷胸汤主治。

Differentiation of pulse and syndrome / pattern [related to] taiyang disease and treatment (part 3)

【英译】

Line 135

Cold damage, six or seven days [after occurrence], [characterized by] chest bind, excess-heat, sunken and tight pulse, pain beneath the heart as hard as stone, [should be] treated by Da Xianxiong Decoction (大陷胸汤, major decoction for resolving chest sinking).

【英译】

Line 136

About ten more days [after occurrence of] cold damage, [there are] heat binding in the internal and alternate chilliness and heat. [It can be] treated by Da Chaihu Decoction (大柴胡汤, major bupleurum decoction). [If there is] just chest bind, but no exuberate heat, it is [caused by] retention of water in the chest and costal region. [If there is just] slight sweating over the head, it [can be] treated by Da Xianxiong Decoction (大陷胸汤, major decoction for resolving chest sinking).

【原文】

(一三七)

太阳病,重发汗而复下之,不大便五六日,舌上燥而渴,日晡所小有潮热,从心下至少腹鞭满而痛,不可近者,大陷胸汤主之。

【今译】

太阳病,经过多次发汗又再次用攻下法治疗,患者有五六日没有大便,舌上干燥而口渴,午后至傍晚体内有微微的潮热,从心下至少腹部坚硬、胀满而疼痛,手不敢触摸,宜用大陷胸汤主治。

【原文】

(一三八)

小结胸病,正在心下,按之则痛,脉浮滑者,小陷胸汤主之。

小陷胸汤方

黄连一两、半夏半升(洗)、栝楼实大者一枚。

右三味,以水六升,先煮栝楼,取三升,去滓,内诸药,煮取两升,去滓,分温三服。

【今译】

小结胸病,正位于心下胃脘部,以手按之则疼痛,脉象浮滑,宜用小陷胸汤主治。

Differentiation of pulse and syndrome/pattern [related to] taiyang disease and treatment（part 3）

【英译】

Line 137

［If］ taiyang disease with repeated perspiration ［is treated］ repeatedly by purgation，［it will result in］ no defecation in five to six days，dryness of tongue and thirst，slight tidal fever in the late afternoon，hardness and fullness from the heart to the lower abdomen with untouchable pain. ［It can be］ treated by Da Xianxiong Decoction （大陷胸汤，major decoction for resolving chest sinking）.

【英译】

Line 138

Minor chest bind disease ［located］ below the heart ［is characterized by］ pain under pressure and floating and slippery pulse，［which can be］ treated by Xiao Xianxiong Decoction（小陷胸汤，minor decoction for resolving chest sinking）.

Xiao Xianxiong Decoction （小陷胸汤，minor decoction for resolving chest sinking）［is composed of］ 1 *liang* of Huanglian（黄连，coptis，Rhizoma Coptidis），0. 5 *sheng* of Banxia （半夏，pinellia，Rhizoma Pinelliae）（washed）and 1 big piece of Gualoushi （栝楼实，trichosanthes，Fructus Trichosanthes）.

These three ingredients are decocted in 6 *sheng* of water. Gualoushi（栝楼实，trichosanthes，Fructus Trichosanthes）is boiled first to get 3 *sheng* ［after］ boiling. ［After］ removal of dregs，other ingredients are put into ［it］ and boiled to get 2 *sheng* ［after］ boiling. ［After］ removal of dregs，［the decoction］ is divided into 3 doses and taken warm.

【原文】

(一三九)

太阳病,二三日,不能卧,但欲起,心下必结,脉微弱者,此本有寒分也,反下之,若利止,必作结胸;未止者,四日复下之,此作协热利也。

【今译】

太阳病发作两三天后,患者不能平卧,只想坐起,心下痞结胀硬,脉象微弱,这是素有寒结的缘故。治疗时如果反而用攻下法,必然导致腹泻。如果腹泻停止,结胸就会出现。如果腹泻没有停止,到了第四天再行攻下,就会引起协热利。

【原文】

(一四〇)

太阳病,下之,其脉促,不结胸者,此为欲解也;脉浮者,必结胸;脉紧者,必咽痛;脉弦者,必两胁拘急;脉细数者,头痛未止;脉沉紧者,必欲呕;脉沉滑者,协热利;脉浮滑者,必下血。

【今译】

太阳病,用攻下法治疗,患者的脉象就会急促,但未有结胸症状,这是邪欲外解的征象。脉象浮的,结胸必然发作。脉象紧的,咽痛必然发生。脉象弦的,两胁必然拘急。脉细数的,头痛还未停止。脉沉紧的,必有欲呕之状。脉沉滑的,将会出现协热下利之症。脉浮滑的,必有大便下血。

Differentiation of pulse and syndrome/pattern [related to] taiyang disease and treatment (part 3)

【英译】

Line 139

Taiyang disease, two or three days [after occurrence], [is characterized by] inability to lie supinely, desire to sit, bind beneath the heart, thin and weak pulse. Originally [there is] cold [in this disease]. [When treated] by purgation, [it will cause diarrhea]. If diarrhea ceases, chest bind must occur. [If diarrhea] does not cease [and is treated] again by purgation in the fourth day, diarrhea mixed with heat will occur.

【英译】

Line 140

[If] taiyang disease [is treated by] purgation, the pulse [will become] speedy, [but there is] no chest bind, [indicating that the disease is] about to resolve. [If] the pulse is floating, there must be chest bind; [if] the pulse is tight, there must be sore-throat; [if] the pulse is taut, there must be intercostals spasm; [if] the pulse is thin and rapid, headache will not stop; [if] the pulse is sunken and tight, there must be nausea; [if] the pulse is sunken and slippery, there must be diarrhea mixed with heat; [if] the pulse is floating and slippery, there must be bloody stool.

【原文】

(一四一)

病在阳,应以汗解之。反以冷水潠之,若灌之,其热被劫不得去,弥更益烦,肉上粟起,意欲饮水,反不渴者,服文蛤散。若不差者,与五苓散。寒实结胸,无热证者,与三物小陷胸汤,白散亦可服。

文蛤散方

文蛤五两。

右一味为散,以沸汤和一升温服,汤用五合。

五苓散方

猪苓十八铢(去黑皮)、白术十八铢、泽泻一两六铢、茯苓十八铢、桂枝半两(去皮)。

上五味,捣为散。白饮和方寸匕服之,每日三服,多饮暖水,汗出愈。

白散方

桔梗三分、巴豆一分(去皮心,熬黑,研如脂)、贝母三分。

右三味为散,内巴豆,更于臼中杵之,以白饮和服,强人半钱匕,

Differentiation of pulse and syndrome/pattern [related to] taiyang disease and treatment (part 3)

【英译】

Line 141

Disease in yang (the external) should be resolved by perspiration. [If] cold water is sprayed and poured [for eliminating heat], heat [will be] stagnated and cannot be eliminated, [leading to] severe heat, vexation, cutaneous papules and desire to drink water but no thirst, [which can be treated by] taking Wenge Powder (文蛤散, meretrix clam shell powder). If [the disease] is not cured, Wuling Powder (五苓散, powder made of five medicinal herbs) [can be used to treat it]. [If there is] chest bind with cold-excess but no heat syndrome/pattern, Xiao Xianxiong Decoction (小陷胸汤, minor decoction for resolving chest sinking) with three medicinals [can be used to treat it], Bai Powder (白散, white powder) also [can be] used [to treat it].

Wenge Powder (文蛤散, meretrix clam shell powder) [is composed of] 5 *liang* of Wenge (文蛤, meretrix clam shell, Concha Meretricis) [which is pounded into] powder and boiled into 1 sheng decoction. [The decoction is] taken 5 *ge* [each time].

Wuling Powder (五苓散, powder made of five medicinal herbs) [is composed of] 18 *zhu* of Zhuling (猪苓, polyporus, Polyporus) with black peel removed, 18 *zhu* of Baizhu (白术, rhizome of largehead atractylodes, Rhizoma Atractylodis Macrocephalae) 1 *liang* and 6 *zhu* of Zexie (泽泻, alisma, Rhizoma Alismatis), 18 *zhu* of Fuling (茯苓, poria, Poria) and 0.5 *liang* of Guizhi (桂枝, cinnamon twig, Ramulus Cinnamomi) with bark removed.

These five ingredients are pounded into powder. [The powder is] taken 1 *fangcunbi* (about 1 gram) with water [each time], three times a day. [It is necessary] to drink more warm water [in order to promote

赢者减之。病在膈上必吐,在膈下必利,不利,进热粥一杯,利过不止,进冷粥一杯。身热皮粟不解,欲引衣自覆者,若以水潠之洗之,益令热劫不得出,当汗而不汗则烦,假令汗出已,腹中痛,与芍药三两,如上法。

【今译】

病在表,应通过发汗解表去邪,但因反而用冷水喷洒浇洗之法退热,热邪虽然被水饮冲击但却不能解除,甚至使热更甚,导致烦躁,皮肤出现鸡皮疙瘩,虽然想喝水,但又不口渴,可服用文蛤散治疗。如果服药后仍不愈,可用五苓散治疗。有寒实结胸,但无热症表现的,可用三物小陷胸汤治疗,也可用白散治疗。

Differentiation of pulse and syndrome / pattern
[related to] taiyang disease and treatment（part 3）

sweating]. [When] sweating [is induced, the disease will] heal.

Bai Powder（白散，white powder）[is composed of] 3 *fen* of Jiegeng（桔梗，platycodon grandiflorum，Radix Platycodonis），1 *fen* of Badou（巴豆，croton tiglium，Fructus Crotonis）[which] is boiled black and pounded like fat with bark removed and 3 *fen* of Beimu（贝母，bulb of fritillary，Bulbus Fritillariae Thunbergii）.

These three ingredients are poundered into powder. Badou（巴豆，croton tiglium，Semen Crotonis）is put into [it for the purpose of] pounding in the cauldron. [The powder is] taken with water. Strong person [can take] a half *qianbi* [of the powder each time]. Weak person takes less. [If] the disease [is located] in the diaphragm, there must be vomiting; [if the disease is located] below the diaphragm, there must be diarrhea. [If there is] no diarrhea, one cup of hot porridge [should be taken]. [If] diarrhea continues, one cup of cold porridge [should be taken]. [If there is] fever and skin nodules are not relieved, [the patient] wants to cover his body with clothes. If water [is used to] pour and wash [the body], heat [will be] stagnated and cannot be relieved. [If] diaphoresis [is used] but no sweating [is induced], [the patient will feel] dysphoric. Suppose perspiration is induced [but there is still] pain in the abdomen, 3 *liang* of Shaoyao（芍药，peony，Radix Paeoniae）is added and used in the same way mentioned above.

【原文】

(一四二)

太阳与少阳并病,头项强痛,或眩冒,时如结胸,心下痞鞕者,当刺大椎第一间、肺俞、肝俞,慎不可发汗。发汗则谵语,脉弦,五日谵语不止,当刺期门。

【今译】

太阳与少阳两经同时发病,出现头痛项强,或眩晕昏冒,时而如结胸状,心下痞塞硬结的,应通过针刺大椎、肺俞、肝俞治疗,千万不能用发汗法。误用发汗法就会出现谵语、脉弦,如果经过五天谵语仍然不止的,应通过针刺期门进行治疗。

【原文】

(一四三)

妇人中风,发热恶寒,经水适来,得之七八日,热除而脉迟身凉,胸胁下满,如结胸状,谵语者,此为热入血室也。当刺期门,随其实而取之。

【今译】

妇人患中风证,有发热恶寒之症,正值月经到来。七八天后,热退,脉迟,身凉,胸胁下胀满,像结胸症状一样,同时又谵语,这是热邪进入血室所致,应当通过针刺期门穴以祛除实邪。

Differentiation of pulse and syndrome / pattern [related to] taiyang disease and treatment (part 3)

【英译】

Line 142

Disease involving both taiyang and shaoyang, [characterized by] stiffness and pain of the head and neck, or dizziness, occasional chest bind and lump below the heart, [can be treated by] needling Dazhui (GV 14), Feishu (BL 13) and Ganshu (BL 18). Cares [should be taken] to avoid perspiration. Perspiration [due to wrong treatment will cause] delirium and taut pulse. [If] delirium does not cease [after] five days [of treatment], Qimen (LR 14) should be needled.

【英译】

Line 143

[When] a woman [suffers from] wind stroke, [there are symptoms and signs of] fever and aversion to cold. Menstruation happens to occur. Seven or eight days [after occurrence of the disease], heat is eliminated, the pulse is slow [and there are symptoms and signs of] general coldness and fullness below the chest and rib-side like chest bind and delirium, [indicating that] heat has entered the blood chamber (uterus). Qimen (LR 14) [can be] needled to resolve it.

【原文】

(一四四)

妇人中风,七八日续得寒热,发作有时,经水适断者,此为热入血室。其血必结,故使如疟状,发作有时,小柴胡汤主之。

【今译】

妇人中风,七八天过后,继续出现发热、怕冷等定时发作的症状,月经恰好中止,这是热入血室所致。因邪热内入血室,必与血相结,因而表现如疟疾,宜用小柴胡汤主治。

【原文】

(一四五)

妇人伤寒,发热,经水适来,昼日明了,暮则谵语,如见鬼状者,此为热入血室,无犯胃气及上二焦,必自愈。

【今译】

妇人患伤寒证,身体发热,正值月经到来之时,白天神志清楚,晚间昏聩谵语,此为热入血室所致,不能用损伤胃气及上二焦的方药治疗,其会自动痊愈。

Differentiation of pulse and syndrome / pattern [related to] taiyang disease and treatment (part 3)

【英译】

Line 144

[When] a woman [suffers from] wind stroke, there are [symptoms and signs of] periodic coldness and heat [after] seven or eight days [of occurrence]. [If] menstruation happens to cease, [it] indicates that heat has entered the blood chamber (uterus). [When heat has entered the blood chamber (uterus), it will] mix with the blood, [resulting in periodic fever and aversion to cold] just like malaria occurring at regular time. Xiao Chaihu Decoction (小柴胡汤, minor bupleurium decoction) [can be used] to treat it.

【英译】

Line 145

[When] a woman [suffers from] cold damage with fever during the time of menstruation, [her mind is] clear in the daytime, but [there is] delirium at night like seeing a ghost, indicating that heat has entered the blood chamber (uterus) but will not attack stomach qi and double energizer. [It will] certainly heal naturally.

【原文】

(一四六)

伤寒六七日，发热，微恶寒，支节烦疼，微呕，心下支结，外证未去者，柴胡桂枝汤主之。

柴胡桂枝汤方

桂枝一两半(去皮)、黄芩一两半、人参一两半、甘草一两(炙)、半夏二合半(洗)、芍药一两半、大枣六枚(擘)、生姜一两半(切)、柴胡四两。

右九味，以水七升，煮取三升，去滓，温服一升。本云人参汤，作如桂枝法，加半夏、柴胡、黄芩，复如柴胡法。今用人参做半剂。

【今译】

伤寒病发作六七天后，患者身体发热，微有恶寒，四肢关节烦疼，微微作呕，心下结聚，表证尚未解除，宜用柴胡桂枝汤主治。

Differentiation of pulse and syndrome/pattern [related to] taiyang disease and treatment (part 3)

【英译】

Line 146

Cold damage [disease], six or seven days [after occurrence], [is characterized by] fever, mild aversion to cold, vexing pain of limb joints, slight nausea, stiffness and bind below the heart. [If] the external syndrome/pattern is not relieved, Chaihu Guizhi Decoction (柴胡桂枝汤, bupleurium decoction) [can be used] to treat it.

Chaihu Guizhi Decoction (柴胡桂枝汤, bupleurium decoction) [is composed of] 1.5 *liang* of Guizhi (桂枝, cinnamon twig, Ramulus Cinnamomi) (bark removed), 1.5 *liang* of Huangqin (黄芩, scutellaria, Radix Scutellariae), 1.5 *liang* of Renshen (人参, ginseng, Radix Ginseng), 1 *liang* of Gancao (甘草, licorice, Radix Gylyrrhizae Praeparata) broiled, 2.5 *ge* of Banxia (半夏, pinellia, Rhizoma Pinelliae) (washed), 1.5 *liang* of Shaoyao (芍药, peony, Radix Paeoniae), 6 pieces of Dazao (大枣, jujube, Fructus Ziziphus Jujubae) (broken), 1.5 *liang* of Shengjiang (生姜, fresh ginger, Rhizoma Zingiberis Recens) (cut) and 4 *liang* of Chaihu (柴胡, bupleurum, Bupleuri).

These nine ingredients [are decocted] in 7 *sheng* of water and get 3 *sheng* [after] boiling. [The decoction, after] removal of dregs, is taken 1 *sheng* warm [each time]. The old edition says that Renshen Decoction (人参汤, ginseng decoction) is used [in the same way] as Guizhi Decoction (桂枝汤, cinnamon twig decoction). [When] added with Banxia (半夏, pinellia, Rhizoma Pinelliae), Chaihu (柴胡, bupleurum, Bupleuri) and Huangqin (黄芩, scutellaria, Radix Scutellariae), [it is used in the same way] as Chaihu [Decoction] (柴胡汤, bupleurium decoction). Now Renshen (人参, ginseng, Radix Ginseng) is used as half of the decoction.

【原文】

(一四七)

伤寒五六日,已发汗而复下之,胸胁满微结,小便不利,渴而不呕,但头汗出,往来寒热,心烦者,此为未解也。柴胡桂枝干姜汤主之。

柴胡桂枝干姜汤方

柴胡半斤、桂枝三两(去皮)、干姜二两、栝楼根四两、黄芩三两、牡蛎二两(熬)、甘草二两(炙)。

右七味,以水一斗二升,煮取六升,再煎取三升,温服一升,日三服。初服微烦,复服汗出便愈。

【今译】

伤寒病发作五六天后,已经发汗又再用泻下法治疗,引起胸胁满闷微有硬结,小便不利,口渴,不呕,头部出汗,寒热往来,心中烦躁不安,这是病未除的原因,宜用柴胡桂枝干姜汤主治。

Differentiation of pulse and syndrome/pattern [related to] taiyang disease and treatment (part 3)

【英译】

Line 147

[If] cold damage [disease], five or six days [after occurrence], [is treated by] purgation again [when there is] already perspiration, [it will cause] fullness and slight bind in the chest and rib-side, dysuria, thirst without nausea, sweating over the head, alternate cold and heat and vexation. Chaihu Guizhi Ganjiang Decoction (柴胡桂枝干姜汤, bupleurum, cinnamon twig and dried ginger decoction) [can be used] to treat it.

Chaihu Guizhi Ganjiang Decoction (柴胡桂枝干姜汤, bupleurum, cinnamon twig and dried ginger decoction) [is composed of] 0.5 *jin* of Chaihu (柴胡, bupleurum, Bupleuri), 3 *liang* of Guizhi (桂枝, cinnamon twig, Ramulus Cinnamomi) with bark removed, 2 *liang* of Ganjiang (干姜, dried ginger, Rhizoma Zingiberis), 4 *liang* of Gualougen (栝楼根, trichosanthes root, Radix Trichosanthes), 3 *liang* of Huangqin (黄芩, scutellaria, Radix Scutellariae), 2 *liang* of Muli (牡蛎, oyster shell, Concha Ostreae) boiled and 2 *liang* of Gancao (甘草, licorice, Radix Gylyrrhizae Praeparata) fried.

These seven ingredients are decocted in 1 *dou* and 2 *sheng* of water and to get 6 *sheng* [after] boiling. [After] removal of dregs, [it is] boiled again and get 3 *sheng*. [Each time] 1 *sheng* is taken warm and three times a day. [When] the decoction is taken first, [there will be] mild vexation. [When it] is taken again, [there will be] sweating. [Sweating is helpful for] healing [the disease].

【原文】

(一四八)

伤寒五六日,头汗出,微恶寒,手足冷,心下满,口不欲食,大便鞕,脉细者,此为阳微结,必有表,复有里也。脉沉,亦在里也。汗出,为阳微。假令纯阴结,不得复有外证,悉入在里,此为半在里半在外也。脉虽沉紧,不得为少阴病。所以然者,阴不得有汗,今头汗出,故知非少阴也,可与小柴胡汤。设不了了者,得屎而解。

【今译】

伤寒病发作五六天后,症状表现为头部出汗,微感畏寒,手足逆冷,心下胀满,不想进食,大便坚硬。脉象细,此为阳微结症,必然既有表症又有里症。脉象沉,主病在里。汗出是阳微结的表现。如果是纯阴结症,不应该再有表症,因为病邪已完全入里,此属于半里半表证。脉虽然沉紧,但却不是少阴病的表现,因为阴症不应有汗出。现今头部汗出,所以知道这不是少阴病,可用小柴胡汤治疗。如果服用小柴胡汤后仍不能解,可通大便,大便一通,病即痊愈。

Differentiation of pulse and syndrome/pattern [related to] taiyang disease and treatment (part 3)

【英译】

Line 148

Cold damage [disease], five or six days [after occurrence], [is characterized by] sweating over the head, slight aversion to cold, cold hands and feet, fullness below the heart, no appetite, hard stool and thin pulse. It is mild yang bind with both external and internal [symptoms and signs]. Sunken pulse [indicates that the disease is] in the internal. Sweating [is the manifestation of] mild yang [bind]. If it is pure yin bind, there should be no external syndrome/pattern, and all [the pathogenic factors should have already] entered the internal. Such [a syndrome/pattern] is semi-internal and semi-external. Though the pulse is sunken and tight, it is not shaoyin disease. The reason is that yin [syndrome/pattern] should have no sweating. Now there is sweating over the head, indicating that it is not shaoyin [disease] and Xiao Chaihu Decoction (小柴胡汤, minor bupleurum decoction) [can be used] to treat [it]. [If the disease] is not resolved, [measures can be taken to promote defecation]. [When] defecation is normalized, [the disease will be] cured.

【原文】

(一四九)

伤寒五六日,呕而发热者,柴胡汤证具,而以他药下之,柴胡证仍在者,复与柴胡汤。此虽已下之,不为逆,必蒸蒸而振,却发热汗出而解。若心下满而鞕痛者,此为结胸也。大陷胸汤主之。但满而不痛者,此为痞,柴胡不中与之,宜半夏泻心汤。

半夏泻心汤方

半夏半升(洗),黄芩、干姜、人参、甘草(炙)各三两,黄连一两,大枣十二枚(擘)。

右七味,以水一斗,煮取六升,去滓,再煎取三升,温服一升,日三服。须大陷胸汤者,方用前第二法。一方用半夏一升。

【今译】

伤寒发作五六日后,临床表现为呕逆而且发热,柴胡汤证的症候已经具备,若用其他攻下方药治疗,但只要柴胡证仍存在,就可继续用柴胡汤治疗。虽然已经误用攻下法治疗了,但也不是逆候,必然出现高热战栗之相,但发热汗出就能使病得解。假如攻下后发生心下胀满而硬痛的,此为结胸症,可用大陷胸汤治疗。如果心下只闷满而不疼痛的,此为痞证,柴胡汤不适合使用,宜用半夏泻心汤治疗。

Differentiation of pulse and syndrome/pattern [related to] taiyang disease and treatment (part 3)

【英译】

Line 149

[In] cold damage [disease], five or six days [after occurrence], [if there are] nausea and fever, [the symptoms and signs of] Chaihu Decoction (柴胡汤, bupleurium decoction) [syndrome/pattern] are already present and [can be treated by] purgation with other medicinals. [But if] Chaihu Decoction (柴胡汤, bupleurum decoction) [syndrome/pattern] is still present, Chaihu Decoction (柴胡汤, bupleurum decoction) still can be used [to treat it]. Although purgation is used, it is not an adverse [treatment]. [When Chaihu Decoction (柴胡汤, bupleurium decoction) is used,] there must be feverish and quivering. [It is just because there are] fever and sweating, [the disease is] cured. If there are fullness, stiffness and pain below the heart, it is chest bind and Da Xianxiong Decoction (大陷胸汤, major decoction for resolving chest sinking) [can be used] to treat it. But [if there is] fullness without pain, it is lump. [To treat such a disease,] Chaihu [Decoction] (柴胡汤, bupleurum decoction) is not suitable, Banxia Xiexin Decoction (半夏泻心汤, pinellia decoction for draining the heart) is appropriate.

Banxia Xiexin Decoction (半夏泻心汤, pinellia decoction for draining the heart) [is composed of] 0.5 *sheng* of Banxia (半夏, pinellia, Rhizoma Pinelliae) (washed), 3 *liang* of Huangqin (黄芩, scutellaria, Radix Scutellariae), 3 *liang* of Ganjiang (干姜, dried ginger, Rhizoma Zingiberis), 3 *liang* of Renshen (人参, ginseng, Radix Ginseng), 3 *liang* of Gancao (甘草, fried licorice, Radix Gylyrrhizae Praeparata) (broiled), 1 *liang* of Huanglian (黄连, coptis, Rhizoma Coptidis), and 12 pieces of Dazao (大枣, jujube, Fructus Ziziphus Jujubae) (broken).

These seven ingredients are decocted in 1 *dou* of water to get 6 *sheng* [after] boiling. [After] removal of dregs, [it is] boiled again to get 3 *sheng*. [The decoction is] taken 1 *sheng* warm [each time] and three times a day. [If] Da Xianxiong Decoction (大陷胸汤, major decoction for resolving chest sinking) is needed, [it can be used according to] the second method mentioned previously. 1 sheng of Banxia (半夏, pinellia, Rhizoma Pinelliae) is need [for the decoction].

【原文】

(一五〇)

太阳、少阳并病,而反下之,成结胸;心下鞭,下利不止,水浆不下,其人心烦。

【今译】

太阳与少阳并病,如果反而用攻下法治疗,必然引起结胸,出现心下硬结,腹泻不止,汤水不能下咽,烦躁不安等症状。

【原文】

(一五一)

脉浮而紧,而复下之,紧反入里,则作痞,按之自濡,但气痞耳。

【今译】

脉象浮而紧,如误用下法治之,脉象浮紧则变为沉紧,会引起痞症。按之柔软,因为仅是气痞而已。

【原文】

(一五二)

太阳中风,下利,呕逆,表解者,乃可攻之。其人漐漐汗出,发作有时,头痛,心下痞鞭满,引胁下痛,干呕,短气,汗出不恶寒者,此表解里未和也,十枣汤主之。

Differentiation of pulse and syndrome/pattern [related to] taiyang disease and treatment（part 3）

【英译】

Line 150

[If] the disease involving both taiyang and shaoyang [is treated by] purgation，[it will cause] chest bind，[leading to] stiffness below the heart，repeated diarrhea，difficulty to drink water and vexation.

【英译】

Line 151

[If the disease with] floating and tight pulse [is treated by] purgation，[floating and] tight [pulse will] change into sunken [pulse] and [there will appear] lump felt soft because it is qi lump.

【英译】

Line 152

Taiyang [disease with] wind stroke [is characterized by] diarrhea and nausea. [If] the external [syndrome/pattern is already] relieved，purgation still [can be used] to treat it. [When] the patient [has] slight sweating at fixed time [and suffers from] headache，lump，stiffness and pain below the heart，pain under the rib-side，dry retching，shortness of breath，sweating and no aversion to cold，it [indicates that] the external [syndrome/pattern] is resolved but the internal is not harmonized. [Then] Shizao Decoction（十枣汤，ten jujubes decoction）[can be used] to treat it.

Shizao Decoction（十枣汤，ten jujubes decoction）[is composed of] Yuanhua（芫花，genkwa，Flos Genkwa）（simmered），Gansui（甘遂，

十枣汤方

芫花（熬）、甘遂、大戟、大枣十枚。

右三味，等分，各别捣为散，以水一升半，先煮大枣肥者十枚，取八合，去滓，内药末，强人服一钱匕，羸人服半钱，温服之，平旦服。若下少，病不除者，明日更服，加半钱，得快下利后，糜粥自养。

【今译】

太阳中风，症见腹泻，呕逆等，治疗时应当先解表。解表后才能使用攻下法攻逐水饮。如果患者微微出汗，定时而发，头痛，心下痞结胀硬，牵引胁下疼痛，干呕，短气，汗出不恶寒的，这是表已解而里未和的缘故，宜用十枣汤主治。

【原文】

（一五三）

太阳病，医发汗，遂发热，恶寒，因复下之，心下痞，表里俱虚，阴阳气并竭，无阳则阴独，复加烧针，因胸烦，面色青黄，肤𥉻者，难治。今色微黄，手足温者，易愈。

【今译】

太阳病，医生若用发汗法治疗，患者汗后仍然发热畏寒，于是医生又再次用攻下法治疗，引起心下痞满，表里均虚，阴阳之气同时耗竭，表症已无，里症独存。医生如果再用烧针法治疗，引发患者心胸烦躁不安，面色青黄、筋肉战栗，为难治之证。如果患者面色微黄、手足温暖，则易治愈。

Differentiation of pulse and syndrome/pattern
[related to] taiyang disease and treatment (part 3)

kansui, Radix Kansui), Daji (大戟, euphorbia, Radix Euphorbiae Pekinesis) and 10 pieces of Dazao (大枣, jujube, Fructus Ziziphus Jujubae).

These three ingredients are equal in dosage, pounded separately into powder and put in 1.5 *sheng* of water. Ten pieces of Dazao (大枣, jujube, Fructus Ziziphus Jujubae) [that are] plump are boiled first to get 8 *ge* of water. [Then] dregs are removed and powder is put into it. A strong person can take 1 *qianbi* (about 1 gram) while a weak person can take a half of *qianbi* (about 0.5 gram). [The decoction should be] taken warm in the morning. If defecation is little and the disease is not eliminated, [it should be] taken again the next day and a half of *qianbi* (about 0.5 gram) [should be] increased [to each dose]. [When] defecation is normal and smooth, [the patient should take] rice porridge to nourish himself.

【英译】

Line 153

Taiyang disease [treated by] diaphoresis will cause fever and aversion to cold. [If treated] again by purgation, [it will lead to] lump below the heart, dual deficiency of the external and internal, exhaustion of yin qi and yang qi, and no yang (external syndrome/pattern) only yin (internal syndrome/pattern). [If treated] again [by acupuncture with] heated needle, [it will cause] thoracic vexation, bluish and yellowish complexion and muscular spasm, [which is] difficult to treat. Now the skin is slightly yellow, the hands and feet are warm, [it is] easy to cure.

【原文】

(一五四)

心下痞,按之濡,其脉关上浮者,大黄黄连泻心汤主之。

大黄黄连泻心汤方

大黄二两、黄连一两。

右二味,以麻沸汤二升渍之,须臾,绞去滓,分温再服。

【今译】

患者心下痞塞,但按之柔软,关部脉象浮,宜用大黄黄连泻心汤治疗。

【原文】

(一五五)

心下痞,而复恶寒汗出者,附子泻心汤主之。

附子泻心汤方

大黄二两、黄连一两、黄芩一两、附子一枚(炮,去皮,破,别煮取汁)。

右四味,切三味,以麻沸汤二升渍之,须臾绞去滓,内附子汁,分温再服。

【今译】

心下痞满,又再次出现恶寒汗出等症状,宜用附子泻心汤主治。

Differentiation of pulse and syndrome/pattern [related to] taiyang disease and treatment (part 3)

【英译】

Line 154

[When there is] lump below the heart [that is] soft under pressure and floating pulse in the guan region, [it can be] treated by Dahuang Huanglian Xiexin Decoction (大黄黄连泻心汤, rhubarb and coptis decoction for draining the heart).

Dahuang Huanglian Xiexin Decoction (大黄黄连泻心汤, rhubarb and coptis decoction for draining the heart) [is composed of] 2 *liang* of Dahuang (大黄, rhubarb, Radix et Rhizoma Rhei) and 1 *liang* of Huanglian (黄连, coptis, Rhizoma Coptidis).

These two ingredients are soaked in 2 *sheng* of boiled water for a whole. [After] a while and removal of the dregs, [it is] divided [into two doses] and taken warm.

【英译】

Line 155

[When there is] lump below the heart with aversion to cold and sweating, Fuzi Xiexin Decoction (附子泻心汤, aconite decoction for draining the heart) [can be used] to treat it.

Fuzi Xiexin Decoction (附子泻心汤, aconite decoction for draining the heart) [is composed of] 2 *liang* of Dahuang (大黄, rhubarb, Radix et Rhizoma Rhei), 1 *liang* of Huanglian (黄连, coptis, Rhizoma Coptidis), 1 *liang* of Huangqin (黄芩, scutellaria, Radix Scutellariae) and 1 piece of Fuzi (附子, aconite, Radix Aconiti Lateralis Preparata) (fry heavily, remove the bark, break, and boil separately to get juice).

These four ingredients, [among which] three are cut first, are decocted in 2 *sheng* of boiled water. [After] a while, the dregs are removed and aconite juice is put into it. [The decoction] is divided [into two doses] and taken warm.

【原文】

(一五六)

本以下之,故心下痞,与泻心汤,痞不解,其人渴而口燥,烦,小便不利者,五苓散主之。

【今译】

本来因为误用了下法,导致心下痞满,可用泻心汤治疗,但痞满却不能解除,且患者口干燥、心烦、小便不畅,宜用五苓散主治。

【原文】

(一五七)

伤寒汗出,解之后,胃中不和,心下痞鞕,干噫食臭,胁下有水气,腹中雷鸣,下利者,生姜泻心汤主之。

生姜泻心汤方

生姜四两(切)、甘草三两(炙)、人参三两、干姜一两、黄芩三两、半夏半升(洗)、黄连一两、大枣十二枚(擘)。

右八味,以水一斗,煮取六升,去滓,再煎取三升,温服一升,日三服。附子泻心汤,本云加附子,半夏泻心汤,甘草泻心汤,同体别名耳。生姜泻心汤,本云理中人参黄芩汤去桂枝术加黄连。并泻肝法。

Differentiation of pulse and syndrome / pattern [related to] taiyang disease and treatment (part 3)

【英译】

Line 156

Because of original [application of] purgation, [there is] a lump below the heart. [When treated by] Xiexin Decoction (泻心汤, decoction for draining the heart), the lump is not relieved and the patient feels thirsty with dryness of the mouth, vexation and dysuria. Wuling Powder (五苓散, powder made of five medicinal herbs) [can be used] to treat it.

【英译】

Line 157

Cold damage [disease], after sweating and relief [of the external], [characterized by] disharmony of the stomach, lump and stiffness below the heart, dry belching with malodor of food, water qi (edema) under the rib-side, thunderous borborygmus and diarrhea, [can be] treated by Shengjiang Xiexin Decoction (生姜泻心汤, ginger decoction for draining the heart).

Shengjiang Xiexin Decoction (生姜泻心汤, ginger decoction for draining the heart) [is composed of] 4 *liang* of Shengjiang (生姜, fresh ginger, Rhizoma Zingiberis Recens) (cut), 3 *liang* of Gancao (甘草, fried licorice, Radix Gylyrrhizae Praeparata) (broiled), 3 *liang* of Renshen (人参, ginseng, Radix Ginseng), 1 *liang* of Ganjiang (干姜, dried ginger, Rhizoma Zingiberis), 3 *liang* of Huangqin (黄芩, scutellaria, Radix Scutellariae), 0.5 *sheng* of Banxia (半夏, pinellia, Rhizoma Pinelliae) (washed), 1 *liang* of Huanglian (黄连, coptis, Rhizoma Coptidis) and 12 pieces of Dazao (大枣, jujube, Fructus Ziziphus Jujubae) (broken).

These eight ingredients are decocted in 1 *dou* of water to get 6 *sheng* [after] boiling. [After] removal of the dregs, [it is] boiled again to get 3 *sheng*. [The decoction is] taken warm 1 *sheng* [each time] and three times a day. Fuzi Xiexin Decoction (附子泻心汤, aconite decoction for draining the heart) originally means to add Fuzi (附子, aconite, Radix Aconiti Lateralis Preparata), so Banxia Xiexin Decoction (半夏泻心汤, ginger decoction for draining the heart) and Gancao Xiexin Decoction (甘草泻心汤, licorice decoction for draining the heart) [are] the

【今译】

伤寒病,汗出表解之后,因胃中不和,而致心下痞硬,嗳气,有食臭味,胁下有水气,肠中有雷鸣,腹泻,宜用生姜泻心汤治疗。

【原文】

(一五八)

伤寒中风,医反下之,其人下利,日数十行,谷不化,腹中雷鸣,心下痞鞕而满,干呕,心烦不得安。医见心下痞,谓病不尽,复下之,其痞益甚。此非结热,但以胃中虚,客气上逆,故使鞕也。甘草泻心汤主之。

甘草泻心汤方

甘草四两(炙)、黄芩三两、干姜三两、半夏半升(洗)、大枣十二枚(擘)、黄连一两。

右六味,以水一斗,煮取六升,去滓,再煎取三升,温服一升,日三服。

【今译】

伤寒中风症,医生反而用攻法治疗,导致患者一日腹泻数十次,泻下清谷,腹中肠鸣如雷声,心下痞满硬结,干呕,心中烦躁不安。医生见心下痞硬,以为病邪未尽,又再次使用攻下法,致使痞胀更甚。这种情况并非邪热内结,而是胃中虚弱,浊气上逆,因而使心下痞硬,宜用甘草泻心汤主治。

Differentiation of pulse and syndrome / pattern [related to] taiyang disease and treatment (part 3)

same in composition but different in name. Shengjiang Xiexin Decoction (生姜泻心汤,ginger decoction for draining the heart) originally means to remove Guizhi (桂枝，cinnamon twig, Ramulus Cinnamomi)and add Huanglian (黄连，coptis, Rhizoma Coptidis) to Renshen Huangqin Decoction (人参黄芩汤,ginseng and scutellaria decoction) for purging the liver.

【英译】

Line 158

Cold damage or wind stroke [should be treated by diaphoresis for resolving the external], [if treated by] purgation, [it will make] the patient [suffer from] diarrhea over ten times a day, indigestion, thunderous borborygmus, lump, stiffness and fullness below the heart, dry retching and vexation. Seeing the lump below the heart, the doctor realizes that the disease is not eliminated and uses purgation again [to treat it], making the lump more serious. Such [a disease] is not heat bind, but stomach deficiency [due to] upward counterflow of pathogenic qi, therefore causing hardness [in the epigastric region]. Gancao Xiexin Decoction (甘草泻心汤, licorice decoction for draining the heart) [can be used] to treat it.

Gancao Xiexin Decoction (甘草泻心汤, licorice decoction for draining the heart) [is composed of] 4 *liang* of Gancao (甘草, licorice, Radix Gylyrrhizae Praeparata) (broil), 3 *liang* of Huangqin (黄芩, scutellaria, Radix Scutellariae), 3 *liang* of Ganjiang (干姜, dried ginger, Rhizoma Zingiberis), 0. 5 *sheng* of Banxia (半夏, pinellia, Rhizoma Pinelliae) (washed), 12 pieces of Dazao (大枣, jujube, Fructus Ziziphus Jujubae) (broken) and 1 *liang* of Huanglian (黄连, coptis, Rhizoma Coptidis).

These six ingredients are decocted in 1 *dou* of water to get 6 *sheng* [after] boiling. [After] removal of dregs, [it is] boiled again to get 3 *sheng*. [The decoction is] taken warm 1 *sheng* [each time] and three times a day.

【原文】

（一五九）

伤寒，服汤药，下利不止，心下痞鞕。服泻心汤已，复以他药下之，利不止，医以理中与之，利益甚。理中者，理中焦，此利在下焦，赤石脂禹余粮汤主之。复不止者，当利其小便。

赤石脂禹余粮汤方

赤石脂一斤（碎）、禹余粮一斤（碎）。

右二味，以水六升，煮取两升，去滓，分温三服。

【今译】

伤寒病，服用泻下的汤药后，腹泻依然不止，心下痞胀硬结。用泻心汤治疗后，又再用其他汤药攻下，导致腹泻不止，医生又使用理中汤，使得腹泻更甚。理中汤是治疗因中焦虚寒而引起的腹泻症，而此类腹泻则在于下焦不固，应用赤石脂禹余粮汤主治。如果用赤石脂禹余粮汤治疗后患者腹泻仍然不止的，应用利小便法治疗。

Differentiation of pulse and syndrome/pattern [related to] taiyang disease and treatment (part 3)

【英译】

Line 159

[In treating the external syndrome/pattern of] cold damage [disease], [application of] the decoction [for purgation causes] incessant diarrhea, lump and stiffness below the heart. The doctor has used Xiexin Decoction (泻心汤, decoction for draining the heart) [to treat it] and other medicinals for purgation, failing to cease incessant diarrhea. [To resolve it,] the doctor has used Lizhong Decoction (理中汤, decoction for regulating the middle), making incessant diarrhea more severe. Lizhong Deccotion (理中汤, decoction for regulating the middle) is used to regulate the middle energizer. [In this case,] incessant diarrhea results from [insecurity of] the middle energizer [which can be] treated by Chishizhi Yuyuliang Decoction (赤石脂禹余粮汤, halloysite and limonite decoction). [If diarrhea is] not ceased, [the therapeutic methods for] promoting urination [can be used].

Chishizhi Yuyuliang Decoction (赤石脂禹余粮汤, halloysite and limonite decoction) [is composed of] 1 *jin* of Chishizhi (赤石脂, halloysite, Halloysitum Rubrum) (pound) and 1 *jin* of Yuyuliang (禹余粮, limonite, Limonitum) (pound).

These two ingredients are decocted in 6 *sheng* of water to get 2 *sheng* [after] boiling. [After] removal of dregs, [the decoction is] divided [into three doses] and taken warm.

【原文】

(一六〇)

伤寒吐下后,发汗,虚烦,脉甚微,八九日心下痞鞕,胁下痛,气上冲咽喉,眩冒,经脉动惕者,久而成痿。

【今译】

伤寒症,误用吐下和发汗法治疗后,导致患者心烦不安,脉象非常微弱,病情迁延八九天后,更出现心下痞结胀硬,胁下疼痛,气上冲咽喉,眩晕昏冒,全身经脉振颤,时间久了,就会形成痿症。

【原文】

(一六一)

伤寒发汗,若吐,若下,解后,心下痞鞕,噫气不除者,旋覆代赭汤主之。

旋覆代赭汤方

旋覆花三两、人参二两、生姜五两、代赭石一两、甘草三两(炙)、半夏半升(洗)、大枣十二枚(擘)。

右七味,以水一斗,煮取六升,去滓,再煎取三升,温服一升,日三服。

【今译】

伤寒病,通过发汗,或涌吐或攻下等方法治疗,外邪已解,只有心下痞硬、噫气不除的,宜用旋覆代赭汤治疗。

Differentiation of pulse and syndrome/pattern [related to] taiyang disease and treatment (part 3)

【英译】

Line 160

[When] cold damage [disease is treated by] purgation [for inducing vomiting], [it will cause] sweating, deficiency-vexation, severe faint pulse, lump and stiffness below the heart for eight or nine days, pain under the rib-side, dizziness and jerking of the meridians [all over the body]. Long-term duration will cause wilting.

【英译】

Line 161

[In] cold damage, [when treated by] diaphoresis or purgation and after relief of [external pathogenic factors], [there are still] lump and stiffness below the heart. [If] retching is not eliminated, Xuanfu Daizhe Decoction (旋覆代赭汤, inula and hematite decoction) [can be used] to treat it.

Xuanfu Daizhe Decoction (旋覆代赭汤, inula and hematite decoction) [is composed of] 3 *liang* of Xuanfuhua (旋覆花, inula flower, Flos Inulae), 2 *liang* of Renshen (人参, ginseng, Radix Ginseng), 5 *liang* of Shengjiang (生姜, fresh ginger, Rhizoma Zingiberis Recens), 1 *liang* of Daizheshi (代赭石, hematite, Haematitum), 3 *liang* of Gancao (甘草, fried licorice, Radix Glycyrrhizae Praeparata) broiled, 0.5 *sheng* of Banxia (半夏, pinellia, Rhizoma Pinelliae) washed and 12 pieces of Dazao (大枣, jujube, Fructus Ziziphus Jujubae) broken.

These seven ingredients are decocted in 1 *dou* of water to get 6 *sheng* [after] boiling. [When] dregs are removed, [it is] boiled again to get 3 *sheng*. [The decoction is] taken warm 1 *sheng* [each time] and three times a day.

【原文】

（一六二）

下后，不可更行桂枝汤，若汗出而喘，无大热者，可与麻黄杏仁甘草石膏汤。

【今译】

用攻下法治疗表证后，不能再用桂枝汤治疗，如果出汗且气喘，无大热症状的，可用麻黄杏仁甘草石膏汤治疗。

【原文】

（一六三）

太阳病，外证未除，而数下之，遂协热而利，利下不止，心下痞鞕，表里不解者，桂枝人参汤主之。

桂枝人参汤方

桂枝四两（别切）、甘草四两（炙）、白术三两、人参三两、干姜三两。

右五味，以水九升，先煎四味，取五升，内桂，更煮取三升，去滓，温服一升，日再夜一服。

【今译】

太阳病，外证还未解除，却多次用攻下法治疗，因此就导致挟表热而腹泻的症状。如果腹泻不断，心下痞塞硬满，表证与里证均未解除，宜用桂枝人参汤治疗。

Differentiation of pulse and syndrome/pattern [related to] taiyang disease and treatment (part 3)

【英译】

Line 162

[When the external syndrome/pattern is treated by] purgation, Guizhi Decoction (桂枝汤, cinnamon decoction) cannot be used again. If [there are symptoms and signs of] sweating, panting and absence of severe heat, Mahuang Xingren Gancao Shigao Decoction (麻黄杏仁甘草石膏汤, ephedra, apricot kernel, licorice and gypsum decoction) [can be used] to treat it.

【英译】

Line 163

[In] taiyang disease, [when] external syndrome/pattern is not eliminated, but purgation is repeatedly used, [it will cause] diarrhea mixed with heat. [If] diarrhea is incessant, [there will be] lump and stiffness below the heart. [To deal with] external and internal [syndromes/patterns that are] not resolved, Guizhi Renshen Decoction (桂枝人参汤, cinnamon twig and ginseng decoction) [can be used] to treat it.

Guizhi Renshen Decoction (桂枝人参汤, cinnamon twig and ginseng decoction) [is composed of] 4 *liang* of Guizhi (桂枝, cinnamon twig, Ramulus Cinnamomi) prepared separately and processed separately, 4 *liang* of Gancao (甘草, fried licorice, Radix Glycyrrhizae Praeparata) broiled, 3 *liang* of Baizhu (白术, rhizome of largehead atractylodes, Rhizoma Atractylodis Ovatae), 3 *liang* of Renshen (人参, ginseng, Radix Ginseng) and 3 *liang* of Ganjiang (干姜, dried ginger, Rhizoma Zingiberis).

These five ingredients are decocted in 9 *sheng* of water. The first four ingredients are boiled first to get 5 *sheng*. [Then] Guizhi (桂枝, cinnamon twig, Ramulus Cinnamomi) is put into [it] to boil and get 3 *sheng*. [After] removal of the dregs, [the decoction is] taken 1 *sheng* warm [each time], once in the daytime and again at night.

【原文】

(一六四)

伤寒大下后,复发汗,心下痞,恶寒者,表未解也,不可攻痞,当先解表,表解乃可攻痞,解表宜桂枝汤,攻痞宜大黄黄连泻心汤。

【今译】

伤寒病,用攻下法治疗后,再使用发汗法,就会导致心下痞塞,恶寒,表症未解,不能攻法消痞,而应先解表,表症解除以后才能用攻法消痞。解表宜用桂枝汤,攻下消痞宜用大黄黄连泻心汤。

【原文】

(一六五)

伤寒发热,汗出不解,心中痞鞕,呕吐而下利者,大柴胡汤主之。

【今译】

伤寒发热,出汗而热不退,心中痞硬,呕吐,腹泻,宜用大柴胡汤治疗。

Differentiation of pulse and syndrome/pattern [related to] taiyang disease and treatment（part 3）

【英译】

Line 164

[In] cold damage [disease]，after [application of] purgation and diaphoresis，[it causes] lump below the heart. [If there is] aversion to cold，[it indicates that] external [syndrome/pattern] is not resolved. The lump cannot be attacked first. [What should be done] first is to resolve the external [syndrome/pattern]. Only when the external [syndrome/pattern] is resolved can the lump be attacked. To resolve the external [syndrome/pattern]，Guizhi Decoction（桂枝汤，cinnamon twig decoction）should be used. To attack the lump，Dahuang Huanglian Xiexin Decoction（大黄黄连泻心汤，rhubarb and coptis decoction for draining the heart）should be used.

【英译】

Line 165

Cold damage [disease]，[characterized by] fever，sweating without relieving [heat]，lump and stiffness in the heart，vomiting and diarrhea，[can be] treated by Da Chaihu Decoction（大柴胡汤，major bupleurum decoction）.

【原文】

（一六六）

病如桂枝证，头不痛，项不强，寸脉微浮，胸中痞鞕，气上冲喉咽，不得息者，此为胸有寒也。当吐之，宜瓜蒂散。

瓜蒂散方

瓜蒂一分（熬黄）、赤小豆一分。

右二味，各别捣筛，为散已，合治之，取一钱匕，以香豉一合，用热汤七合，煮作稀糜，去滓，取汁和散，温顿服之。不吐者，少少加，得快吐乃止。诸亡血、虚家，不可与瓜蒂散。

【今译】

疾病的症状像桂枝证，但患者头不痛，项不拘急，寸脉微浮，胸中痞胀硬结，气上冲咽喉，呼吸受阻，这是胸中有寒所致，应当用吐法治疗，宜用瓜蒂散主治。

Differentiation of pulse and syndrome/pattern [related to] taiyang disease and treatment (part 3)

【英译】

Line 166

The disease, [manifested] as cinnamon twig syndrome/pattern, [is characterized by] absence of both headache and stiffness of nape, slight floating of cun pulse, lump and stiffness in the chest and difficult to breathe due to qi surging upward to the throat. It indicates [that there is] cold in the chest and should [be treated by] vomiting [therapy]. Guadi Powder (瓜蒂散, melon stalk powder) is the appropriate [formula].

Guadi Powder (瓜蒂散, melon stalk powder) [is composed of] 1 *fen* of Guadi (瓜蒂, melon stalk, Pedicellus Melo) (simmered yellow) and 1 *fen* of Chixiaodou (赤小豆, rice bean, Semen Phaseoli).

These two ingredients are pounded and sieved separately, making into powder and combined for treatment. 1 *qianbi* (about 1 gram) of mixed powder and 1 *ge* of Xiangchi (香豉, fermented soybean, Sojae Praeparatum) are put into 7 *ge* of hot water to be boiled as porridge. The dregs are removed, the juice and powder are combined. [It is] taken warm as one single dose. [If the patient] does not vomit, add a little more. [When the patient begins] to vomit, cease [taking the powder]. [Those who suffer from] blood collapse and deficiency, Guadi Powder (瓜蒂散, melon stalk powder) cannot be used.

【原文】

(一六七)

病胁下素有痞,连在脐旁,痛引少腹,入阴筋者,此名脏结,死。

【今译】

病人胁下常有痞块,连及脐旁,疼痛牵引少腹,甚至痛及阴茎,此病称为脏结,为死候。

【原文】

(一六八)

伤寒若吐、若下后,七八日不解,热结在里,表里俱热,时时恶风,大渴,舌上干燥而烦,欲饮水数升者,白虎加人参汤主之。

白虎加人参汤方

知母六两、石膏一斤(碎、绵裹)、甘草二两(炙)、人参二两、粳米六合。

右五味,以水一斗,煮米熟汤成,去滓,温服一升,日三服。此方立夏后、立秋前乃可服,立秋后不可服,正月二月三月尚凛冷,亦不可与服之,与之则呕利而腹痛。诸亡血虚家,亦不可与,得之则腹痛利者,但可温之,当愈。

【今译】

伤寒病,或用吐法或用下法治疗后,七八日后病依然未能解除,患者蕴热于里,表里均热,时时感觉恶风,大渴,舌苔干燥,心烦不安,想喝大量的水,宜用白虎加人参汤治疗。

Differentiation of pulse and syndrome/pattern [related to] taiyang disease and treatment（part 3）

【英译】

Line 167

Under the rib-side of the patient, there is lump extending to the navel and pain involving the lower abdomen and stretching into the penis. This is called visceral bind, [which is] fatal.

【英译】

Line 168

[In] cold damage [disease], [if treated] either by vomiting [therapy] or by purgation [therapy], [after] seven or eight days, [the disease is] not resolved, [and there are symptoms and signs of] heat bind in the internal, heat in both the external and internal, frequent aversion to wind, severe thirst, dryness of the tongue surface, vexation and desire to drink several *sheng* of water. [It can be] treated by Baihu Decoction (白虎汤, white tiger decoction) added with Renshen (人参, ginseng, Ginseng).

Baihu Decoction （白虎汤, white tiger decoction) added with Renshen (人参, ginseng, Ginseng) [is composed of] 6 *liang* of Zhimu (知母, rhizome of common anemarrhena, Rhizoma Anemarrhenae), 1 *jin* of Shigao (石膏, gypsum, Gypsum Fibrosum) broken and gauze wrapped, 2 *liang* of Gancao (甘草, fried licorice, Radix Glycyrrhizae Praeparata) broiled, 2 *liang* of Renshen (人参, ginseng, Radix Ginseng) and 6 *ge* of Jingmi (粳米, polished round-grained rice, Semen Oryzae Sativae).

These five ingredients are decocted in 1 *dou* of water and the rice is boiled thoroughly. The dregs are removed and [the decoction] is taken warm 1 *sheng* [each time] and three times a day. This decoction still can be used after beginning of Summer and before beginning of Autumn. After beginning of Autumn, it cannot be used. [In] January, February and March[of the lunar calendar], [it is] still cold, [this decoction] cannot still be used, otherwise [it will cause] vomiting, diarrhea and abdominal pain. [Those who suffer from] blood collapse and deficiency cannot also be treated by [this decoction], [otherwise it will] cause abdominal pain and diarrhea. But [if the patient] feels warm, [the disease is] about to heal.

【原文】

(一六九)

伤寒无大热,口燥渴,心烦,背微恶寒者,白虎加人参汤主之。

【今译】

伤寒病,患者无大热,口干燥而渴,心中烦躁不安,背部微感恶寒,宜用白虎加人参汤主治。

【原文】

(一七〇)

伤寒,脉浮,发热,无汗,其表不解,不可与白虎汤。渴欲饮水,无表证者,白虎加人参汤主之。

【今译】

伤寒病,患者脉象浮,发热,无汗,此为表证未解,不可用白虎汤治疗。如果口渴想喝水,表证已除,宜用白虎加人参汤治疗。

Differentiation of pulse and syndrome／pattern [related to] taiyang disease and treatment（part 3）

【英译】

Line 169

Cold damage [disease], [characterized by] absence of great heat, dryness of mouth, thirst, vexation and slight aversion to cold in the back, [should be] treated by Baihu Decoction（白虎汤, white tiger decoction）added with Renshen（人参, ginseng, Ginseng）.

【英译】

Line 170

Cold damage [disease], [characterized by] floating pulse, fever and absence of sweating, [indicates that] the external [syndrome/pattern] is not resolved and cannot be treated by Baihu Decoction（白虎汤, white tiger decoction）. [If the patient feels] thirsty and wants to drink water, [it indicates that] the external [syndrome/pattern] is absent and can be treated by Baihu Decoction（白虎汤, white tiger decoction）added with Renshen（人参, ginseng, Ginseng）.

【原文】

(一七一)

太阳、少阳并病,心下鞕,颈项强而眩者,当刺大椎、肺俞、肝俞,慎勿下之。

【今译】

太阳少阳并病,患者有心下痞结胀硬,颈项拘急,头晕目眩等症状,应针刺大椎、肺俞、肝俞治疗,而攻下之法不可使用。

【原文】

(一七二)

太阳与少阳合病,自下利者,与黄芩汤。若呕者,黄芩加半夏生姜汤主之。

黄芩汤方

黄芩三两、芍药二两、甘草二两(炙)、大枣十二枚(擘)。

右四味,以水一斗煮取三升,去滓,温服一升,日再,夜一服。

【今译】

太阳与少阳并病,患者有自动腹泻的,用黄芩汤治疗。如有呕吐的,用黄芩加半夏生姜汤治疗。

Differentiation of pulse and syndrome / pattern [related to] taiyang disease and treatment (part 3)

【英译】

Line 171

[The disease] involving taiyang and shaoyang, [characterized by] hardness below the heart, stiffness of the neck and nape, and dizziness, should [be treated by] needling Dazhui (GV 14), Feishu (BL 13) and Ganshu (BL 18). Purgation cannot be used.

【英译】

Line 172

Disease involving both taiyang and shaoyang, [marked by] spontaneous diarrhea, [can be] treated by Huangqin Decoction (黄芩汤, scutellaria decoction). If there is retching, [it can be] treated by Huangqin Decoction (黄芩汤, scutellaria decoction) added with Banxia (半夏, pinellia, Rhizoma Pinelliae) and Shengjiang (生姜, fresh ginger, Rhizoma Zingiberis Recens).

Huangqin Decoction (黄芩汤, scutellaria decoction) [is composed of] 3 *liang* of Huangqin (黄芩, scutellaria, Radix Scutellariae), 2 *liang* of Shaoyao (芍药, peony, Radix Paeoniae), 2 *liang* of Gancao (甘草, fried licorice, Radix Glycyrrhizae Praeparata) broiled and 12 pieces of Dazao (大枣, jujube, Fructus Ziziphus Jujubae) broken.

These four ingredients are decocted in 1 *dou* of water to get 3 *sheng* [after] boiling. [After] removal of the dregs, [the decoction is] taken warm 1 *sheng* [each time], twice in the daytime and once at night.

【原文】

（一七三）

伤寒，胸中有热，胃中有邪气，腹中痛，欲呕吐者，黄连汤主之。

黄连汤方

黄连三两、甘草三两（炙）、干姜三两、桂枝三两（去皮）、人参二两、半夏半升（洗）、大枣十二枚（擘）。

右七味，以水一斗，煮取六升，去滓，温服，昼三，夜二。疑非仲景方。

【今译】

伤寒病，患者胸脘部有热，胃中有邪气，腹中疼痛，想呕吐，宜用黄连汤主治。

Differentiation of pulse and syndrome/pattern [related to] taiyang disease and treatment (part 3)

【英译】

Line 173

Cold damage [disease], [characterized by] heat in the chest, pathogenic factors in the stomach, abdominal pain and desire to vomit, [should be] treated by Huanglian Decoction (黄连汤, coptis decoction).

Huanglian Decoction (黄连汤, coptis decoction) [is composed of] 3 *liang* of Huanglian (黄连, coptis, Rhizoma Coptidis), 3 *liang* of Gancao (甘草, fried licorice, Radix Glycyrrhizae Praeparata) broiled, 3 *liang* of Ganjiang (干姜, dried ginger, Rhizoma Zingiberis), 3 *liang* of Guizhi (桂枝, cinnamon twig, Ramulus Cinnamomi) bark-removed, 2 *liang* of Renshen (人参, ginseng, Radix Ginseng), 0. 5 *sheng* of Banxia (半夏, pinellia, Rhizoma Pinelliae) washed and 12 pieces of Dazao (大枣, jujube, Fructus Ziziphus Jujubae) broken.

These seven ingredients are decocted in 1 *dou* of water to get 6 *sheng* [after] boiling. [After] removal of the dregs, [the decoction is] taken warm, thrice in the daytime and twice at night. Perhaps this decoction was not formulated by Zhang Zhongjing.

【原文】

(一七四)

伤寒八九日,风湿相搏,身体疼烦,不能自转侧,不呕,不渴,脉浮虚而涩者,桂枝附子汤主之。若其人大便鞕,小便自利者,去桂加白术汤主之。

桂枝附子汤方

桂枝四两(去皮)、附子三枚(炮,去皮,破)、生姜三两(切)、大枣十二枚(擘)、甘草二两(炙)。

右五味,以水六升,煮取二升,去滓,分温三服。

去桂加白术汤方

附子三枚(炮,去皮,破)、白术四两、生姜三两(切)、甘草二两(炙)、大枣十二枚(擘)。

右五味,以水六升,煮取二升,去滓,分温三服,初一服,其人身如痹,半日许复服之,三服都尽。其人如冒状,勿怪,此以附子、术并走皮内,逐水气未得除,故使之耳,法当加桂四两,此本一方二法,以大便硬,小便自利,去桂也;以大便不硬,小便不利,当加桂,附子三枚恐多也,虚弱家及产妇,宜减服之。

Differentiation of pulse and syndrome / pattern [related to] taiyang disease and treatment（part 3）

【英译】

Line 174

Cold damage [disease], eight or nine days [after occurrence], [is characterized by] conflict between wind and dampness, general vexing pain, difficulty in turning the body, no retching and no thirst as well as floating, weak and rough pulse. [It should be] treated by Guizhi Fuzi Decoction（桂枝附子汤, cinnamon twig and aconite decoction）. If there are hard stool and spontaneous urination, the decoction with removal of Guizhi（桂枝, cinnamon twig, Ramulus Cinnamomi）and addition of Baizhu（白术, rhizome of largehead atractylodes, Rhizoma Atractylodis Macrocephalae）[can be used] to treat it.

Guizhi Fuzi Decoction（桂枝附子汤, cinnamon twig and aconite decoction）[is composed of] 4 *liang* of Guizhi（桂枝, cinnamon twig, Ramulus Cinnamomi）bark-removed, 3 pieces of Fuzi（附子, aconite, Radix Aconiti Lateralis Preparata）（fry heavily, remove the peel and break）, 3 *liang* of Shengjiang（生姜, fresh ginger, Rhizoma Zingiberis Recens）cut, 12 pieces of Dazao（大枣, jujube, Fructus Ziziphus Jujubae）broken and 2 *liang* of Gancao（甘草, licorice, Radix Glycyrrhizae Praeparata）broiled.

These five ingredients are decocted in 6 *sheng* of water to get 2 *sheng* [after] boiling. [After] removal of the dregs, [the decoction is] divided [into three doses] and taken warm.

Decoction with removal of Guizhi（桂枝, cinnamon twig, Ramulus Cinnamomi）and addition of Baizhu（白术, rhizome of largehead atractylodes, Rhizoma Atractylodis Macrocephalae）[is composed of] 3 pieces of Fuzi（附子, aconite, Radix Aconiti Lateralis Preparata）（fry heavily, remove the peel and break）, 4 *liang* of Baizhu（白术, rhizome of largehead atractylodes, Rhizoma Atractylodis Macrocephalae）, 3 *liang* of Shengjiang（生姜, fresh

【今译】

伤寒病发作八九天后，风湿相互搏结，患者出现身体疼痛，烦躁，不能自行侧转，不作呕，口不渴，脉象浮虚而涩等症状，宜用桂枝附子汤主治。如果患者大便硬结、小便通畅，则宜用去桂加白术汤主治。

Differentiation of pulse and syndrome / pattern [related to] taiyang disease and treatment (part 3)

ginger, Rhizoma Zingiberis Recens) cut, 2 *liang* of Gancao (甘草, licorice, Radix Glycyrrhizae Praeparata) broiled and 12 pieces of Dazao (大枣, jujube, Fructus Ziziphus Jujubae) broken.

These five ingredients are decocted in 6 *sheng* of water to get 2 *sheng* [after] boiling. [After] removal of dregs, [the decoction is] divided into three doses and taken warm. [If after] taking the first [dose, the patient feels] like [having] impediment [in the whole] body, [another dose can be] taken in about half a day. [After] taking all the three [doses], the patient seems to be dizzy. [It is] not strange, [because] Fuzi (附子, aconite, Radix Aconiti Lateralis Preparata) and Baizhu (白术, rhizome of largehead atractylodes, Rhizoma Atractylodis Macrocephalae) have penetrated beneath the skin, failing to expel water qi (dampness due to water retention). That is why [dizziness occurs]. The therapeutic method [used to treat it is] to add 4 *liang* of Guizhi (桂枝, cinnamon twig, Ramulus Cinnamomi). This formula [can be used in] two ways: if [there are symptoms and signs of] hard stool and spontaneously normal urination, Guizhi (桂枝, cinnamon twig, Ramulus Cinnamomi) is removed; if stool is not hard and urination is not spontaneously normal, Guizhi (桂 枝, cinnamon twig, Ramulus Cinnamomi) should be added. 3 pieces of Fuzi (附子, aconite, Radix Aconiti Lateralis Preparata), [in some cases], may be too much. For weak patients and lying-in women, it is appropriate to take less [of the decotion].

【原文】

（一七五）

风湿相搏，骨节疼烦，掣痛不得屈伸，近之则痛剧，汗出短气，小便不利，恶风不欲去衣，或身微肿者，甘草附子汤主之。

甘草附子汤方

甘草二两（炙）、附子二枚（炮，去皮，破）、白术二两、桂枝四两（去皮）。右四味，以水六升，煮取三升，去滓，温服一升，日三服。初服得微汗则解。能汗止复烦者，将服五合。恐一升多者，宜服六七合为始。

【今译】

风湿相互搏结，骨关节疼痛，烦躁，牵引拘急，不能屈伸，按之则疼痛更甚，汗出，短气，小便不畅，恶风，不愿脱衣，或者身体轻微浮肿，宜用甘草附子汤主治。

Differentiation of pulse and syndrome / pattern [related to] taiyang disease and treatment (part 3)

【英译】

Line 175

[The disease, characterized by] conflict between wind and dampness, vexing pain of joints [that makes it] difficult to bend and stretch [the limbs], pain [that is] exacerbated under pressure, sweating, shortness of breath, dysuria, aversion to cold without desire to put off clothes, or slight swelling of the body, [should be] treated by Gancao Fuzi Decoction (甘草附子汤, licorice and aconite decoction).

Gancao Fuzi Decoction (甘草附子汤, licorice and aconite decoction) [is composed of] 2 *liang* of Gancao (甘草, fried licorice, Radix Glycyrrhizae Praeparata) broiled, 2 pieces of Fuzi (附子, aconite, Radix Aconiti Lateralis Preparata) (fry heavily, remove the peel and break), 2 *liang* of Baizhu (白术, rhizome of largehead atractylodes, Rhizoma Atractylodis Macrocephalae) and 4 *liang* of Guizhi (桂枝, cinnamon twig, Ramulus Cinnamomi) (remove the bark).

These four ingredients are decocted in 6 *sheng* of water to get 3 *sheng* [after] boiling. [After] removal of the dregs, [the decoction is] taken warm 1 *sheng* [each time] and three times a day. [If] there is slight sweating [after] the first [time of] taking [the decoction], [it indicates that the disease is] eliminated. [If after the first time of taking the decoction, the patient is] able to eat, perspiration ceases, but vexation returns, 6 *ge* [of the decoction] should be taken. [If] 1 *sheng* [for the first dose is felt] too much, 6 or 7 *ge* is appropriate.

【原文】

(一七六)

伤寒,脉浮滑,此以表有热,里有寒,白虎汤主之。

白虎汤方

知母六两、石膏一斤(碎)、甘草二两(炙)、粳米六合。

右四味,以水一斗,煮米熟,汤成,去滓,温服一升,日三服。

【今译】

伤寒病,脉象浮滑,表有热,里有寒,宜用白虎汤主治。

Differentiation of pulse and syndrome / pattern [related to] taiyang disease and treatment (part 3)

【英译】

Line 176

[In] cold damage [disease], [if there is] floating and slippery pulse, it [indicates that] there is heat in the external and cold in the internal. Baihu Decoction (白虎汤, white tiger decoction) [is used] to treat it.

Baihu Decoction (白虎汤, white tiger decoction) [is composed of] 6 *liang* of Zhimu (知母, anemarrhena, Rhizoma Anemarrhenae), 1 *jin* of Shigao (石膏, gypsum, Gypsum) (break), 2 *liang* of Gancao (甘草, fried licorice, Radix Glycyrrhizae Praeparata) broiled and 6 *ge* of Jingmi (粳米, polished round-grained rice, Semen Oryzae sativae).

These four ingredients are decocted in 1 *dou* of water. [When] the rice is well cooked, the decoction is perfect. [After] removal of the dregs, [the decoction is] taken warm 1 *sheng* [each time] and three times a day.

【原文】

(一七七)

伤寒，脉结代，心动悸，炙甘草汤主之。

炙甘草汤方

甘草四两(炙)、生姜三两(切)、人参二两、生地黄一斤、桂枝三两(去皮)、阿胶二两、麦门冬半升(去心)、麻仁半升、大枣三十枚(擘)。

右九味，以清酒七升，水八升，先煮八味，取三升，去滓，内胶烊消尽，温服一升，日三服。一名复脉汤。

【今译】

伤寒病，脉象结代，心悸不宁，宜用炙甘草汤主治。

Differentiation of pulse and syndrome / pattern [related to] taiyang disease and treatment (part 3)

【英译】

Line 177

Cold damage [disease], [characterized by] binding-intermittent pulse and palpitation, [should be] treated by Zhigancao Decoction (炙甘草汤, fried licorice decoction).

Zhigancao Decoction (炙甘草汤, fried licorice decoction) [is composed of] 2 *liang* of Gancao (甘草, licorice, Radix Glycyrrhizae Praeparata) (broil), 3 *liang* of Shengjiang (生姜, fresh ginger, Rhizoma Zingiberis Recens) (cut), 2 *liang* of Renshen (人参, ginseng, Radix Ginseng), 1 *jin* of Shengdihuang (生地黄, fresh rehmannia, Radix Rehmanniae), 3 *liang* of Guizhi (桂枝, cinnamon twig, Ramulus Cinnamomi) (remove the bark), 2 *liang* of Ejiao (阿胶, ass-hide glue, Colla Corii Asini), 0.5 *sheng* of Maimendong (麦门冬, ophiopogon, Radix Ophiopogonis), 0.5 *sheng* of Maren (麻仁, hemp seed, Fructus Cannabis) and 30 pieces of Dazao (大枣, jujube, Fructus Ziziphus Jujubae) (break).

These nine ingredients are put in 7 *sheng* of clear wine and 8 *sheng* of water. Eight ingredients are boiled to get 3 *sheng*. [After] removal of the dregs, Ejiao (阿胶, ass-hide glue, Colla Corii Asini) is put into it [to boil till it is] completely melted. [The decoction is] taken warm 1 *sheng* [each time] and three times a day. [This decoction] is also called Fumai Decoction (复脉汤, decoction for normalizing the beating of pulse).

【原文】

(一七八)

脉按之来缓,时一止复来者,名曰结。又脉来动而中止,更来小数,中有还者反动,名曰结,阴也;脉来动而中止,不能自还,因而复动者,名曰代,阴也。得此脉者,必难治。

【今译】

脉象按之则缓,时而停止,但又继续搏动的,名为结脉。又有脉象跳动时突然中止,更有微数之相,脉搏停止间歇时间短,还能复跳,这种脉象称为"结",属于阴脉。脉象跳动中突然停止,但不能自还,因而继续再搏动,这种脉象称为"代",属于阴脉。有这种脉象的,都很难治疗。

Differentiation of pulse and syndrome / pattern [related to] taiyang disease and treatment (part 3)

【英译】

Line 178

[If] the pulse appears moderate under pressure, now ceasing and then beating, it is called binding. [If] the pulse now beats and then ceases, during [which it may] turn normal, it is called binding of yin [in nature]. [If] the pulse now beats and then ceases, [during which it] cannot turn normal and starts to beat [after a certain period of time], it is called intermittent [pulse] of yin [in nature]. [The patient] with such a pulse is difficult to cure.

辨阳明病脉证并治

【原文】

(一七九)

问曰：病有太阳阳明，有正阳阳明，有少阳阳明，何谓也？答曰：太阳阳明者，脾约是也；正阳阳明者，胃家实是也；少阳阳明者，发汗、利小便已，胃中燥、烦、实，大便难是也。

【今译】

问：病有太阳阳明、有正阳阳明、有少阳阳明等三种情况，各指的是什么呢？

答：太阳阳明证，指的是脾约证。正阳阳明证，指的是胃家实证。少阳阳明证，指的是误用发汗、利小便之法而导致的胃中干燥、烦躁、邪实，大便因此而难的病症。

【原文】

(一八〇)

阳明之为病，胃家实是也。

【今译】

阳明病的机理，就是胃肠燥实。

Differentiation of pulse and syndrome / pattern
〔related to〕 yangming disease and treatment

Differentiation of pulse and syndrome/pattern [related to] yangming disease and treatment

【英译】

Line 179

Question: A disease may have 〔three kinds of syndromes/patterns〕, either taiyang and yangming, or zhengyang and yangming, or shaoyang and yangming. What is the reason?

Answer: Taiyang and yangming 〔syndrome/pattern〕 indicates spleen restriction; zhengyang and yangming 〔syndrome/pattern〕 indicates stomach excess; shaoyang and yangming 〔syndrome/pattern〕 indicates dryness, vexatioin and excess in the stomach 〔due to treatment for〕 promoting perspiration and urination, causing difficulty in defecation.

【英译】

Line 180

〔The pathogenesis of〕 the disease of yangming is stomach excess.

【原文】

(一八一)

问曰：何缘得阳明病？答曰：太阳病，若发汗，若下，若利小便，此亡津液，胃中干燥，因转属阳明。不更衣，内实，大便难者，此名阳明也。

【今译】

问：阳明病是怎么发生的呢？

答：患太阳病的病人，如果发汗太过，或误用攻下法，或误用利小便法治疗，就会导致津液损伤，肠胃干燥，病邪因而传入阳明，出现大便不解、肠胃燥结成实、大便困难等症状，这就是所谓的阳明病。

【原文】

(一八二)

问曰：阳明病外证云何？答曰：身热，汗自出，不恶寒，反恶热也。

【今译】

问：阳明病的外在症候是怎么样的呢？

答：主要表现为患者身热，汗自出，不恶寒，反而恶热。

Differentiation of pulse and syndrome/pattern [related to] yangming disease and treatment

【英译】

Line 181

Question: What is the cause of yangming disease?

Answer: [In] taiyang disease, if sweating is profuse, purgation [is wrongly used] and [treatment for] promoting urination [is also wrongly used], it [will lead to] loss of fluid and humor and dryness in the stomach. [Consequently pathogenic factors will] transmit into yangming. [If there appear] constipation, internal excess and difficulty in defecation, it is called yangming [disease].

【英译】

Line 182

Question: What are the characteristics of external syndrome/pattern of yangming disease?

Answer: [They are] fever, spontaneous sweating, no aversion to cold but aversion to heat.

【原文】

(一八三)

问曰：病有得之一日，不发热而恶寒者，何也？答曰：虽得之一日，恶寒将自罢，即自汗出而恶热也。

【今译】

问：患病的第一天，患者不发热而恶寒，原因是什么呢？

答：虽然是患病的第一天，恶寒也会自行停止，很快就会自然出汗而恶热。

【原文】

(一八四)

问曰：恶寒何故自罢？答曰：阳明居中，主土也。万物所归，无所复传。始虽恶寒，二日自止，此为阳明病也。

【今译】

问：恶寒症状为什么会自了呢？

答：阳明为中，属土，土为万物所归之处，没有什么能够再传。虽然患者刚开始恶寒，但第二日自会停止，这就是阳明病。

Differentiation of pulse and syndrome/pattern [related to] yangming disease and treatment

【英译】

Line 183

Question: In the first day of [yangming] disease, [there is] no fever but aversion to cold. What is the reason?

Answer: Although this is the first day of [yangming disease], aversion to cold will spontaneously cease, and [there will certainly be] spontaneous sweating and aversion to heat soon.

【英译】

Line 184

Question: Why aversion to cold spontaneously ceases?

Answer: [The reason is that] yangming is located in the center, governing the earth [where] all things converge and nothing will transmit. Although [there is] aversion to cold at the beginning, [it will] spontaneously cease the next day. This is [the manifestation] of yangming disease.

【原文】

(一八五)

本太阳,初得病时,发其汗,汗先出不彻,因转属阳明也。伤寒发热,无汗,呕不能食,而反汗出濈濈然者,此转属阳明也。

【今译】

本来属太阳病,刚发病的时候,使用了发汗法治疗。由于出汗不透彻,因而使邪气内传阳明经。伤寒病有发热、无汗、呕吐、不能进食等症状。如果反而出现不断出汗的症状,就是邪传阳明的表现。

【原文】

(一八六)

伤寒三日,阳明脉大。

【今译】

伤寒病发作的第三日,病传入阳明。脉象则大。

Differentiation of pulse and syndrome / pattern [related to] yangming disease and treatment

【英译】

Line 185

Originally [it is] taiyang disease. At the beginning [of the disease], [treatment of] diaphoresis [is used]. [Because] perspiration is not thorough, [pathogenic factors] transmit to yangming. [In] cold damage [disease], [the symptoms and signs of] fever, absence of perspiration, retching without ability to eat and repeated sweating [indicate that pathogenic factors] have transmitted to yangming.

【英译】

Line 186

On the third day of cold damage [disease], [the disease is located in] yangming and the pulse is large.

【原文】

(一八七)

伤寒脉浮而缓,手足自温者,是为系在太阴。太阴者,身当发黄,若小便自利者,不能发黄。至七八日,大便鞕者,为阳明病也。

【今译】

伤寒病,脉象浮而缓,手足温暖的,病属太阴。太阴寒湿内郁,患者身体应发黄。若小便通畅的,则不会发黄。到了第七天或第八天,若大便硬结,为湿邪化燥,说明已转成阳明病。

【原文】

(一八八)

伤寒转系阳明者,其人濈然微汗出也。

【今译】

伤寒由他经转为阳明病的,病人将连绵不断地微微出汗。

*Differentiation of pulse and syndrome／pattern
［related to］yangming disease and treatment*

【英译】

Line 187

［In］ cold damage ［disease］, ［the symptoms and signs of］ floating and moderate pulse ［as well as］ warm hands and feet indicate ［it］ is in taiyin. ［In］ taiyin ［disease］, ［the patient's］ body should be yellow. If there is spontaneous urination, ［the body］ is not yellow. Hard stool, seven or eight days ［after occurrence of the disease, indicates that it］ is yangming disease.

【英译】

Line 188

［When pathogenic factors in］ cold damage ［disease］ have transmitted to yangming, ［the patient］ will repeatedly have slight sweating.

【原文】

(一八九)

阳明中风,口苦咽干,腹满微喘,发热恶寒,脉浮而紧。若下之,则腹满、小便难也。

【今译】

阳明感受风邪,出现口苦、咽喉干燥、腹部胀满、微微气喘、发热怕冷、脉象浮紧症状的,不能攻下。若误行攻下,则使腹部胀满,小便不易解出。

【原文】

(一九〇)

阳明病,若能食,名中风;不能食,名中寒。

【今译】

阳明病,如果能食,则称为中风;如果不能食,则称为中寒。

Differentiation of pulse and syndrome/pattern [related to] yangming disease and treatment

【英译】

Line 189

Wind stroke in yangming [is characterized by] bitterness in the mouth, dryness of the throat, abdominal fullness, slight panting, fever, aversion to cold, floating and tight pulse. If [treated by] purgation, [it will] cause abdominal fullness and difficulty in defection.

【英译】

Line 190

[In] yangming disease, if [the patient is] unable to eat, it is called wind stroke; [if the patient is] able to eat, [it is] called cold attack.

【原文】

（一九一）

阳明病，若中寒者，不能食，小便不利，手足濈然汗出，此欲作固瘕，必大便初鞕后溏。所以然者，以胃中冷，水谷不别故也。

【今译】

阳明病若有中寒症，且不能饮食，小便不通畅，手足不断汗出，这是即将形成固瘕的征兆，必然使大便初出干硬，而后稀溏。之所以出现这样的情况，是以为胃中寒冷，不能泌别水谷的原因。

【原文】

（一九二）

阳明病，初欲食，小便反不利，大便自调，其人骨节疼，翕翕如有热状，奄然发狂，濈然汗出而解者，此水不胜谷气，与汗共并，脉紧则愈。

【今译】

阳明病，开始食欲正常，大便通畅，但小便却反而不利。病人感到骨节疼痛，似乎有翕翕发热的状况，又突然狂躁不安，不断出汗，病则随之解除。这是水湿不胜谷气的缘故，湿随出汗，脉象变紧，病即愈。

Differentiation of pulse and syndrome/pattern [related to] yangming disease and treatment

【英译】

Line 191

[In] yangming disease, [the symptoms and signs of] cold attack, inablility to eat, dysuria and repeated sweating over hands and feet [indicate that] there will be foxed conglomeration and stool hard first and then sloppy. The reason [is that there is] cold in the stomach, [resulting in] stool with undigested food.

【英译】

Line 192

[In] yangming disease, initially [there is] desire to eat, but urination is unsmooth while defecation is normal. [The patient suffers from] pain of joints, feverish sensation like having heat and sudden mania. [But when there is] repeated sweating,[the disease is] resolved. It [indicates that] water (dampness) cannot overcome cereal qi [and thus] slips out together with perspiration. [When] the pulse becomes tight, [the disease will be] cured.

【原文】

(一九三)

阳明病,欲解时,从申至戌上。

【今译】

阳明病,将解的时间是从申时(15—17 点)到戌时(19—21 点)之间。

【原文】

(一九四)

阳明病,不能食,攻其热必哕,所以然者,胃中虚冷故也。以其人本虚,攻其热必哕。

【今译】

阳明病,不能进食,若采用祛热之法治之,则必然产生呃逆。原因是胃中有虚寒。由于病人本来胃气虚,用苦寒泄热必使胃气更虚,因而产生呃逆。

Differentiation of pulse and syndrome/pattern [related to] yangming disease and treatment

【英译】

Line 193

[The time for] yangming disease to resolve is from shen (15:00 - 17:00) to xu (19:00 - 21:00).

【英译】

Line 194

[In] yangming disease, [the patient is] unable to eat. [If treated by] attacking heat [with cold therapy, it will] inevitably cause hiccup. The reason [is that there is] deficiency-cold in the stomach. Originally the patient is weak, [treatment for] attacking heat [with cold therapy will] certainly cause hiccup.

【原文】

(一九五)

阳明病,脉迟,食难用饱,饱则微烦头眩,必小便难,此欲作谷瘅。虽下之,腹满如故。所以然者,脉迟故也。

【今译】

阳明病,脉迟,进食不能过饱,饱食则会导致微烦不适,头晕眼花,小便必然困难,谷疸将要发作。虽然采用泻下方药,但腹部胀满却依然如故。之所以会产生这种情况,是因为脉迟所致。

【原文】

(一九六)

阳明病,法多汗,反无汗,其身如虫行皮中状者,此以久虚故也。

【今译】

阳明病,应该多汗,但却无汗,病人皮下似乎有虫蠕动。这是长期虚弱所致。

Differentiation of pulse and syndrome/pattern [related to] yangming disease and treatment

【英译】

Line 195

[In] yangming disease, the pulse is slow [and the patient] does not overeat. [If the patient has] overeaten, [it will cause] slight vexation, dizziness and difficulty in defecation, [eventually] leading to grain jaundice (jaundice due to indigestion). Although purgation [is used], abdominal fullness [is still the same] as before. The reason is that the pulse is slow.

【英译】

Line 196

[In] yangming disease, there should be profuse sweating, but in fact there is no sweating and there seems to have worms moving beneath the skin. This is due to long-term deficiency.

【原文】

(一九七)

阳明病,反无汗而小便利,二三日呕而欬,手足厥者,必苦头痛;若不欬、不呕、手足不厥者,头不痛。

【今译】

阳明病,不但无汗,而且小便正常。发病第二、三天的时候,病人作呕又咳嗽,手足厥冷,必然遭受头痛。如果病人不咳嗽,不作呕,手足不厥冷,头就不痛。

【原文】

(一九八)

阳明病,但头眩,不恶寒,故能食而咳,其人咽必痛;若不咳者,咽不痛。

【今译】

阳明病,如果病人头眩但不恶寒,用食时就会咳嗽,其咽喉必然疼痛。如果病人不咳嗽,咽喉就不会痛。

Differentiation of pulse and syndrome / pattern [related to] yangming disease and treatment

【英译】

Line 197

[In] yangming disease, [if there is] absence of sweating and urination is smooth, two or three days [after occurrence, there will be] retching, cough and reversal [cold] of hands and feet. [As a result, the patient will] suffer from headache. If there are [symptoms and signs of] no retching, cough and reversal cold of limbs, [the patient will not] suffer from headache.

【英译】

Line 198

[In] yangming disease, if [there is] dizziness but no aversion to cold, [the patient] will cough [when] taking food and [suffer from] sore-throat. If [there is] no cough, the throat will not be sore.

【原文】

(一九九)

阳明病,无汗,小便不利,心中懊恼者,身必发黄。

【今译】

阳明病若有无汗、小便不利、心中烦闷等症状,病人身体必然发黄。

【原文】

(二〇〇)

阳明病,被火,额上微汗出,而小便不利者,必发黄。

【今译】

阳明病如果以温火之法治之,则额头有微出汗。如果患者小便不利,则身体必然发黄。

【原文】

(二〇一)

阳明病,脉浮而紧者,必潮热,发作有时,但浮者,必盗汗出。

【今译】

阳明病,脉象若浮而紧,必然引起潮热,且发作有时。如果脉象浮,必然引起盗汗。

Differentiation of pulse and syndrome / pattern [related to] yangming disease and treatment

【英译】

Line 199

[In] yangming disease, [if there are symptoms and signs of] no sweating, dysuria and vexation in the heart, [the patient's] body will become yellow.

【英译】

Line 200

[If] yangming disease is treated by fire [therapy], [there will be] slight sweating over the forehead. If [there is] dysuria, [the patient's body] will become yellow.

【英译】

Line 201

[In] yangming disease, [if] the pulse is floating and tight, there must be tidal fever that occurs periodically. If [the pulse is] floating, there will be night sweating.

【原文】

(二〇二)

阳明病,口燥,但欲漱水,不欲咽者,此必衄。

【今译】

阳明病虽有口腔干燥之症,但患者却只想漱口,不想喝水,必然引起鼻孔出血。

【原文】

(二〇三)

阳明病,本自汗出,医更重发汗,病已差,尚微烦不了了者,此必大便鞕故也。以亡津液,胃中干燥,故令大便鞕,当问其小便日几行,若本小便日三四行,今日再行,故知大便不久出。今为小便数少,以津液当还入胃中,故知不久必大便也。

【今译】

阳明病,本来患者自然出汗,医生则重用发汗疗法,病症已经缓解,但还有一些微烦不适之处,这必定是因大便干硬所导致的后果。由于出汗过多而耗伤津液,引起胃中干燥,因而使得大便干硬。这时医生应当询问病人一日小便几次,如果患者小便原来一日三四次,而现在一日则只有两次,就可知道大便不久将自然排出。现根据小便次数减少,可推知津液应当还入胃中,所以就能知道不久大便必解。

Differentiation of pulse and syndrome / pattern [related to] yangming disease and treatment

【英译】

Line 202

[In] yangming disease, [though there is] dryness of the mouth, [the patient] just wants to rinse [the mouth], instead of drinking water. [In such a case, there will been] inevitable epistaxis.

【英译】

Line 203

[In] yangming disease, sweating originally is spontaneous. The doctor has tried to promote perspiration. [As a result,] the disease is already alleviated, but there is still slight vexation due to hard stool. Because of profuse sweating, there is dryness in the stomach. That is why there is hard stool. When asking about how many times of urination in a single day, [the doctor gets to know that the patient] originally urinates three to four times a day, but now just twice a day. That is why [the doctor] knows that stool will spontaneously issue soon. Now urination is frequent but urine is scanty because fluid and humor are still in the stomach. That is why [the doctor] knows that [the patient will] defecate soon.

【原文】

(二〇四)

伤寒呕多,虽有阳明证,不可攻之。

【今译】

伤寒病中呕吐剧烈的患者,虽然有阳明证,但治疗时也不能用攻下之法。

【原文】

(二〇五)

阳明病,心下鞕满者,不可攻之。攻之,利遂不止者死,利止者愈。

【今译】

阳明病,胃脘部硬满的患者,不可用泻下方药治疗。误用泻下之法而导致腹泻不止的,有生命危险;如果腹泻停止,则可痊愈。

【原文】

(二〇六)

阳明病,面合色赤,不可攻之。必发热,色黄者,小便不利也。

【今译】

阳明病中,患者满面通红的,不能用攻下之法治疗。误用攻下之法必然引起发热、肌肤发黄、小便不通畅的变症。

Differentiation of pulse and syndrome / pattern [related to] yangming disease and treatment

【英译】

Line 204

[In] cold damage disease with frequent retching, although there is yangming syndrome/pattern, purgation cannot be used.

【英译】

Line 205

[In] yangming disease, [if there is] stiffness and fullness below the heart, [therapy for] attack cannot be used. [Because] attack [therapy] will cause incessant diarrhea and [make the disease] fatal. [If] diarrhea ceases, [the disease will be] healed.

【英译】

Line 206

[In] yangming disease, [the patient with] redness of the whole face cannot [be treated by] attack [therapy]. [Wrong use of attack therapy will] inevitably cause fever, yellow skin and dysuria.

【原文】

(二〇七)

阳明病,不吐,不下,心烦者,可与调胃承气汤。

【今译】

阳明病,患者没有经过催吐法和泻下法的治疗,但依然心烦不安的,可以用调胃承气汤治疗。

【原文】

(二〇八)

阳明病,脉迟,虽汗出不恶寒者,其身必重,短气,腹满而喘,有潮热者,此外欲解,可攻里也。手足濈然汗出者,此大便已鞕也,大承气汤主之。若汗多,微发热恶寒者,外未解也,其热不潮,未可与承气汤。若腹大满不通者,可与小承气汤,微和胃气,勿令致大泄下。

大承气汤方

大黄四两(酒洗)、厚朴半斤(炙,去皮)、枳实五枚(炙)、芒硝三合。

右四味,以水一斗,先煮二物,取五升,去滓,内大黄,更煮取二升,

*Differentiation of pulse and syndrome/pattern
[related to] yangming disease and treatment*

【英译】

Line 207

[In] yangming disease，[the patient is] not [treated by] vomiting [therapy] and purgation [therapy]，[but there is] still vexation. [It can be] treated by Tiaowei Chengqi Decoction（调胃承气汤，decoction for regulating the stomach and harmonizing qi).

【英译】

Line 208

Yangming disease [is usually characterized by] slow pulse，sweating without aversion to cold，heaviness of the body，shortness of breath，abdominal fullness and panting. [If] there is tidal fever，it is external [syndrome/pattern] and will soon be resolved by attacking the internal. [If there is] frequent sweating，it [indicates] hard stool and can be treated by Da Chengqi Decoction （大承气汤，major decoction for harmonizing qi). If there is profuse sweating with mild fever and aversion to cold，[it indicates that] the external [syndrome/pattern] is not resolved and Chengqi Decoction （承气汤，decoction for harmonizing qi) cannot be used if fever is not tidal. If there is severe abdominal fullness，Xiao Chengqi Decoction （小承气汤，minor decoction for harmonizing qi) can be used [to treat it] to mildly harmonize stomach qi，but [cares should be taken] to avoid causing severe diarrhea.

Da Chengqi Deccotion （大承气汤，major decoction for harmonizing qi) [is composed of] 4 *liang* of Dahuang （大黄，rhubarb，Radix et Rhizoma Rhei) washed in the wine，0.5 *jin* of

去滓，内芒硝，更上微火一两沸，分温再服。得下，余勿服。

小承气汤方

大黄四两（酒洗）、厚朴二两（炙，去皮）、枳实三枚大者（炙）。

右三味，以水四升，煮取一升二合，去滓，分温两服。初服汤当更衣，不尔者尽饮之。若更衣者，勿服之。

【今译】

阳明病的常见症状是，脉象迟，汗出而不恶寒，身体沉重，短气，腹部胀满，喘息。如果有潮热，是表证，即可解除，可用攻里之法；如果手足不断出汗，说明大便已经硬结，可用大承气汤主治；如果汗出较多，且轻微发热而恶寒，说明表证未解，若无潮热，就不能用承气汤治疗；如果腹部胀满、大便不通，可用小承气汤轻微泻下以和畅胃气，而大泻之法则不宜使用。

Differentiation of pulse and syndrome/pattern [related to] yangming disease and treatment

Houpo（厚朴，magnolia bark，Cortex Magnoliae Officinalis）broiled and peel-removed，5 pieces of Zhishi（枳实，unripe bitter orange，Fructus Aurantii Immaturus）broiled and 3 *ge* of Mangxiao（芒硝，mirabilite，Natrii Sulfas）.

These four ingredients are decocted in 1 *dou* of water. Two ingredients are boiled first to get 5 *sheng* of water. [After] removal of dregs，Dahuang（大黄，rhubarb，Radix et Rhizoma Rhei）is boiled in it to get 2 *sheng* of water. [Then] Mangxiao（芒硝，mirabilite，Natrii Sulfas）is boiled in it once or twice under mild fire. [The decoction is] divided [into two doses] and taken warm. [When] defecation occurs，[rest of the decoction is] ceased taking.

Xiao Chengqi Decoction（小承气汤，minor decoction for harmonizing qi）[is composed of] 4 *liang* of Dahuang（大黄，rhubarb，Radix et Rhizoma Rhei）(wash in the wine)，2 *liang* of Houpo（厚朴，magnolia bark，Cortex Magnoliae Officinalis）(broil and remove the bark)，3 pieces of Zhishi（枳实，unripe bitter orange，Fructus Aurantii Immaturus）(broil).

These three ingredients are decocted in 4 *sheng* of water to get 1 *sheng* and 2 *ge* [after] boiling. [After] removal of the dregs，[the decoction is] divided [into two doses] and taken warm. [After] taking [the first dose]，[the patient] should defecate. [If there is no defecation,] the whole decoction should be taken. [If the patient] has already defecated，[there is] no need to take [the decoction again].

【原文】

(二〇九)

阳明病,潮热,大便微鞕者,可与大承气汤,不鞕者,不可与之。若不大便六七日,恐有燥屎,欲知之法,少与小承气汤,汤入腹中,转矢气者,此有燥屎也,乃可攻之。若不转矢气者,此但初头鞕,后必溏,不可攻之。攻之必胀满不能食也。欲饮水者,与水则哕。其后发热者,必大便复鞕而少也,以小承气汤和之。不转矢气者,慎不可攻也。

【今译】

阳明病,有潮热,大便稍微硬结的,可用大承气汤治疗。如果大便不硬结,则不能用大承气汤治疗。如果六七天大便不解,恐有燥屎内阻,要想了解情况,可先用少量的小承气汤予以治疗。服药后如果有排气现象,说明有燥屎,可用攻下之法。服药后如果没有排气现象,说明大便初现硬结、之后必有稀溏,不能采用攻下之法。如果使用攻下之法,则会导致腹部胀满,不能进食。想饮水的,饮水后便有呃逆。如果攻下后又出现发热的,大便必定会再次变硬,但量则较少,应用小承气汤调和。屎气没转的,不能采用攻下之法。

Differentiation of pulse and syndrome / pattern [related to] yangming disease and treatment

【英译】

Line 209

[In] yangming disease，[if there are] tidal fever and mild hard stool，[it can be treated by] Da Chengqi Decoction（大承气汤，major decoction for harmonizing qi）. [If stool is] not hard，[this decoction] cannot be used. If there is no defecation for six or seven days，maybe the stool is dry and get stuck in rectum. In order to know [whether it is so]，small amount of Xiao Chengqi Decoction（小承气汤，minor decoction for harmonizing qi）can be used. [If the patient] breaks wind [when] the decoction [is taken] into the abdomen，it [indicates] dry stool [which can be] attacked. If [the patient] does not break wind [after taking the decoction]，it [indicates that] the stool is hard first and then becomes sloppy，[which] cannot be treated by purgation. [If] be treated by purgation，[it will] cause [abdominal] distension，fullness and inability to eat. If [the patient] desires to drink water，[there will be] hiccup [immediately after] drinking water. [If there is] fever after [being treated by purgation]，[it will] inevitably make the stool hard and scanty. [In such a case，] Xiao Chengqi Decoction（小承气汤，minor decoction for harmonizing qi）[can be used] to regulate it. [If there is] no flatus，cares must be taken not to purgation [it].

【原文】

(二一〇)

夫实则谵语,虚则郑声。郑声者,重语也。直视,谵语,喘满者死,下利者亦死。

【今译】

凡为实邪的,多为谵语;凡为虚怯的,多为郑声。所谓郑声,指的是语言重复。如果两眼直视,且有谵语,同时又兼见气喘胀满的,多为死候。如有下利的,也是死候。

【原文】

(二一一)

发汗多,若重发汗者,亡其阳,谵语,脉短者死;脉自和者不死。

【今译】

发汗太过,或重复发汗,阳气则大伤,出现谵语、脉短等症状,属于死候;若脉自行调和,则不属死候。

Differentiation of pulse and syndrome / pattern
[related to] yangming disease and treatment

【英译】

Line 210

[In] excess [case], there is delirium; [in] deficiency [case], there is muttering. Muttering refers to repetitious speech. [If there are symptoms and signs of] staring eyes, delirium, panting and fullness, it is fatal. [If there is] diarrhea, it is also fatal.

【英译】

Line 211

[If there are symptoms and signs of] profuse sweating, or repeated sweating, [it will] severely damage yang. [If] delirium and short pulse [appear], [it is] fatal. [If] the pulse spontaneously normalizes, [it is] not fatal.

【原文】

(二一二)

伤寒,若吐、若下后,不解,不大便五六日,上至十余日,日晡所发潮热,不恶寒,独语如见鬼状。若剧者,发则不识人,循衣摸床,惕而不安,微喘直视,脉弦者生,涩者死。微者,但发热谵语者,大承气汤主之。若一服利,则止后服。

【今译】

伤寒,若以呕吐或攻下之法治之,但并未解除,五六日甚至十多日没有大便,午后无潮热发作,不恶寒,恍惚自语如鬼状。如果病状剧烈,患者不识身边之人,循衣摸床,惊恐不安,微微喘息,双目直视。在这种情况下,脉象弦者可救,脉象涩者不可救。如果病状轻微,但有发热和谵语症状,可用大承气汤治疗。如果首服汤药大便即通畅,汤药就不用再服了。

【原文】

(二一三)

阳明病,其人多汗,以津液外出,胃中燥,大便必鞕,鞕则谵语,小承气汤主之。若一服谵语止者,更莫复服。

【今译】

阳明病,如果病人多汗,为津液外泄所致,胃中干燥,必然引起大便硬结,大便硬则发生谵语,可用小承气汤治之。假使首服汤药后谵语即停止,就不要再服用了。

Differentiation of pulse and syndrome/pattern [related to] yangming disease and treatment

【英译】

Line 212

[In] cold damage, if [the therapy for] vomiting or [the therapy for] purgation is already used but [the disease is] not resolved, [there are symptoms and signs of] no defecation in five or six days or even more than ten days, tidal fever in the afternoon, no aversion to cold and soliloquy like a ghost. If more serious, [the patient is] unable to recognize the people [around him] with floccillation, fear, disquiet, slight panting and staring straight forward. [In this case, if] the pulse is taut, [it] is curable; [if the pulse is] rough, [it is] fatal. [In] mild [cases], [if there are] fever and delirium, [it can be] treated by Da Chengqi Decoction (大承气汤, major decoction for harmonizing qi). If defecation is normal [after] taking [the first dose], [rest of the decoction] ceases taking.

【英译】

Line 213

[In] yangming disease, profuse sweating is caused by fluid and humor issuing outwards, [consequently leading to] dryness in the stomach and hard stool. Hard stool will cause delirium. Xiao Chengqi Decoction (小承气汤, minor decoction for harmonizing qi) [can be used] to treat it. If delirium ceases [after] taking the first [dose], [rest of the decoction] ceases taking.

【原文】

(二一四)

阳明病,谵语,发潮热,脉滑而疾者,小承气汤主之。因与承气汤一升,腹中转气者,更服一升;若不转气者,勿更与之。明日又不大便,脉反微涩者,里虚也,为难治,不可更与承气汤也。

【今译】

阳明病,病人有谵语、潮热和脉象滑疾等症状,可用小承气汤治疗。如果服用了一升小承气汤,病人开始排气,应再服一升。如果病人没有排气,就不要再服用了。如果第二天又无大便,脉象反而微涩,说明里虚,为难治之症,承气汤就更不可用了。

【原文】

(二一五)

阳明病,谵语,有潮热,反不能食者,胃中必有燥屎五六枚也。若能食者,但鞕耳,宜大承气汤下之。

【今译】

阳明病,有谵语,有潮热,但却不能进食的,是胃肠道中有燥屎五六枚。如果患者还能进食,只是大便硬结,可用大承气汤治之。

Differentiation of pulse and syndrome / pattern [related to] yangming disease and treatment

【英译】

Line 214

[In] yangming disease，[if there are symptoms and signs of] delirium，tidal fever and slippery and racing pulse，Xiao Chengqi Decoction（小承气汤，minor decoction for harmonizing qi）[can be used] to treat it. [If after] taking 1 *sheng* of the decoction and there is flatus in the abdomen，[the patient should] take 1 *sheng* again. If there is no flatus，[the decoction should] not be taken again. [In] the next day，[if there is] no defecation and the pulse is faint and rough，[it indicates that there is] deficiency in the internal，[it is] difficult to heat and Xiao Chengqi Decoction（小承气汤，minor decoction for harmonizing qi）cannot be used.

【英译】

Line 215

[In] yangming disease，[if there are symptoms and signs of] delirium，tidal fever and inability to take food，[it indicates that] there are five or six pieces of hard stool in the stomach [and intestines]. If [the patient is] able to take food，but [there is] hard stool，Da Chengqi Decoction（大承气汤，major decoction for harmonizing qi）[can be used] to treat it.

【原文】

（二一六）

阳明病，下血，谵语者，此为热入血室。但头汗出者，刺期门，随其实而泻之，濈然汗出则愈。

【今译】

阳明病，有下血谵语症状者，为热入血室。但有头出汗者，可针刺期门以泄实邪。若患者全身出汗，病则自愈。

【原文】

（二一七）

汗出，谵语者，以有燥屎在胃中，此为风也。须下者，过经乃可下之。下之若早，语言必乱，以表虚里实故也。下之愈，宜大承气汤。

【今译】

出汗而有谵语的，是肠胃中有燥屎阻结、外有太阳中风所致。此症须用泻下之法治疗，但只有表证解除后才能攻下。如果过早攻下，则会导致语言错乱。这是表虚里实所致。用攻之法治疗才会痊愈，可用大承气汤治之。

Differentiation of pulse and syndrome / pattern [related to] yangming disease and treatment

【英译】

Line 216

[In] yangming disease, excretion of blood and delirium indicates heat entering the blood chamber. If there is sweating over the head, [it can be treated by] needling Qimen (LR 14) to drain excess. [If there is] sweating all over the body, [it will] bring recovery.

【英译】

Line 217

Sweating and delirium are caused by dry stool in the stomach [and intestines], indicating wind [stroke]. [It] should [be treated by] purgation. [Only when external syndrome/pattern is] resolved can purgation [be used]. If purgation [is used] earlier, [it will cause] deranged speech due to external deficiency and internal excess. [It can be] cured by purgation. The appropriate [therapy] is Da Chengqi Decoction (大承气汤, major decoction for harmonizing qi).

【原文】

(二一八)

伤寒四五日,脉沉而喘满,沉为在里,而反发其汗,津液越出,大便为难,表虚里实,久则谵语。

【今译】

伤寒病四五日后,患者脉象沉、气喘、胀满。沉脉属病在里,若以发汗之法治之,可致津液随汗越出,大便因而困难。表虚里实若延久,即会发生谵语。

【原文】

(二一九)

三阳合病,腹满,身重,难以转侧,口不仁,面垢,谵语,遗尿。发汗则谵语。下之则额上生汗,手足逆冷。若自汗出者,白虎汤主之。

白虎汤方

知母六两、石膏一斤(碎)、甘草二两(炙)、粳米六合。

右四味,以水一斗,煮米熟汤成,去滓,温服一升,日三服。

【今译】

若太阳、阳明、少阳三经合病,则腹部胀满,身体沉重,转侧困难,口中麻木不仁,面部垢浊,谵语,遗尿。若用发汗之法治疗,会使谵语更甚。若用攻下之法,则会造成额部汗出,四肢冰冷。如果有自汗出,可用白虎汤治疗。

Differentiation of pulse and syndrome/pattern [related to] yangming disease and treatment

【英译】

Line 218

Four or five days [after occurrence of] cold damage, [there are symptoms and signs of] sunken pulse, panting, distension and fullness. Sunken pulse indicates [that the disease is located in] the internal. [If] diaphoresis is used, [it will lead to] outward straying of fluid and humor, making defecation difficult. [If] external deficiency and internal excess maintain for a long time, delirium will be caused.

【英译】

Line 219

In combination disease of three yang (namely, taiyang, yangming and shaoyang), [there are symptoms and signs of] abdominal fullness, body heaviness, difficulty in turning the body, insensitivity of the mouth, grimy face, delirium and enuresis. [If] diaphoresis [is used], [it will] cause delirium. [If] purgation [is used], [it will induce] sweating over the forehead and reversal cold of hands and feet. If there is spontaneous sweating, Baihu Decoction (白虎汤, white tiger decoction) [can be used] to treat it.

Baihu Decoction (白虎汤, white tiger decoction) [is composed of] 6 *liang* of Zhimu (知母, anemarrhena, Rhizoma Anemarrhenae), 1 *jin* of Shigao (石膏, gypsum, Gypsum) broken, 2 *liang* of Gancao (甘草, licorice, Radix Glycyrrhizae Praeparata) broiled and 6 *ge* Jingmi (粳米, polished round-grained rice, Semen Oryzae Sativae).

These four ingredients are decocted in 1 *dou* of water. When the rice is well cooked, the decoction is finished. [After] removal of the dregs, [the decoction is] taken 1 *sheng* warm and three times a day.

【原文】

(二二〇)

二阳并病，太阳证罢，但发潮热，手足漐漐汗出，大便难而谵语者，下之则愈，宜大承气汤。

【今译】

太阳、阳明两经并病，太阳表证已解，但仍发潮热，手足微微出汗，大便难解而有谵语的，攻下则可痊愈，适宜用大承气汤治疗。

【原文】

(二二一)

阳明病，脉浮而紧，咽燥，口苦，腹满而喘，发热汗出，不恶寒，反恶热，身重。若发汗则躁，心愦愦，反谵语。若加温针，必怵惕，烦躁不得眠。若下之，则胃中空虚，客气动膈，心中懊憹，舌上胎者，栀子豉汤主之。

【今译】

阳明病，脉象浮紧，咽部干燥，口苦，腹部胀满而气喘，发热出汗，不恶寒，反恶热，身体沉重。如用发汗之法，则会引起心中烦乱，导致谵语。如用温针治疗，则会引起怵惕，烦躁，不得安眠。如用泻下之法治疗，则会导致胃中空虚，邪气扰动胸膈，引起心中懊憹，若舌上有腻苔，则可用栀子豉汤治疗。

Differentiation of pulse and syndrome/pattern [related to] yangming disease and treatment

【英译】

Line 220

[In the] disease involving double yang (namely taiyang and yangming), taiyang syndrome/pattern is resolved, but [there are still symptoms and signs of] tidal fever, mild sweating over hands and feet, difficult in defecation and delirium. [It can be] cured by purgation. The appropriate [treatment] is Da Chengqi Decoction (大承气汤, major decoction for harmonizing qi).

【英译】

Line 221

[In] yangming disease, [there are symptoms and signs of] floating and tight pulse, dryness of the throat, bitterness in the mouth, abdominal fullness, panting, fever, sweating, no aversion to cold, aversion to heat and body heaviness. [If treated by] diaphoresis, [it will cause] vexation and delirium. If [treated by acupuncture with] warm needle, [it will] inevitably [cause] anxiety, vexation and insomnia. If [treated by] purgation, [it will] cause stomach deficiency, pathogenic qi stirring the diaphragm, anguish in the heart and thick fur on the tongue. Zhizi Chi Decoction (栀子豉汤, gardenia and fermented soybean decoction) [can be used] to treat it.

【原文】

(二二二)

若渴欲饮水,口干舌燥者,白虎加人参汤主之。

白虎加人参汤方

知母六两、石膏一斤(碎)、甘草二两(炙)、粳米六合、人参三两。

右五味,以水一斗,煮米熟汤成,去滓,温服一升,日三服。

【今译】

如果患者口渴想喝水,口干舌燥,可用白虎加人参汤主治。

【原文】

(二二三)

若脉浮,发热,渴欲饮水,小便不利者,猪苓汤主之。

猪苓汤方

猪苓(去皮)、茯苓、泽泻、阿胶、滑石(碎)各一两。

右五味,以水四升,先煮四味,取二升,去滓,内下阿胶烊消,温服七合,日三服。

【今译】

如果有脉浮、发热、口渴想喝水、小便不畅等症状,以猪苓汤主治。

Differentiation of pulse and syndrome/pattern [related to] yangming disease and treatment

【英译】

Line 222

If [the patient feels] thirsty and wants to drink water, [if] the mouth and tongue are dry, Baihu Decoction (白虎汤, white tiger decoction) added with Renshen (人参, ginseng, Ginseng) [can be used] to treat it.

Baihu Decoction (白虎汤, white tiger decoction) added with Renshen (人参, ginseng, Ginseng) [is composed of] 6 *liang* of Zhimu (知母, anemarrhena, Rhizoma Anemarrhenae), 1 *jin* of Shigao (石膏, gypsum, Gypsum) (break), 2 *liang* of Gancao (甘草, licorice, Radix Glycyrrhizae Praeparata) (broil), 6 *ge* of Jingmi (粳米, polished round-grained rice, Semen Oryzae Sativae) and 3 *liang* of Renshen (人参, ginseng, Radix Ginseng).

These five ingredients are decocted in 1 *dou* of water. When the rice is well cooked, the decoction is finished. [After] removal of the dregs, [the decoction is] taken 1 *sheng* warm and three times a day.

【英译】

Line 223

If [the disease is characterized by] floating pulse, fever, thirst with desire to drink water and inhibited urination, Zhuling Decoction (猪苓汤, polyporus decoction) [can be used] to treat it.

Zhuling Decoction (猪苓汤, polyporus decoction) [is composed of] 1 *liang* of Zhuling (猪苓, polyporus, Polyporus Umbellatus) (break the peel), 1 *liang* of Fuling (茯苓, poria, Poria), 1 *liang* of Zexie (泽泻, alisma, Rhizoma Alismatis), 1 *liang* of Ejiao (阿胶, ass-hide glue, Colla Corri Asini) and 1 *liang* of Huashi (滑石, talcum, Talcum) (crush).

These five ingredients are decocted in 4 *sheng* of water. Four ingredients are boiled first to get 2 *sheng*. [When] the dregs are removed, Ejiao (阿胶, ass-hide glue, Colla Corri Asini) is put into it. [The decoction is] taken 7 *ge* warm [each time] and three times a day.

【原文】

(二二四)

阳明病,汗出多而渴者,不可与猪苓汤,以汗多胃中燥,猪苓汤复利其小便故也。

【今译】

阳明病,汗出多而口渴的,不可用猪苓汤治疗,汗多且胸中燥闷。猪苓汤能够通利病人小便,而进一步损伤津液。

【原文】

(二二五)

脉浮而迟,表热里寒,下利清谷者,四逆汤主之。

【今译】

患者脉浮而迟,表热里寒,泄泻完谷不化,可用四逆汤治之。

【原文】

(二二六)

若胃中虚冷,不能食者,饮水则哕。

【今译】

如果胃中虚寒不能进食的,饮水后则会出现干呕。

Differentiation of pulse and syndrome / pattern
[related to] yangming disease and treatment

【英译】

Line 224

[In] yangming disease，[if there is] profuse sweating with thirst，Zhuling Decoction (猪苓汤，polyporus decoction) cannot [be used] to treat it because profuse sweating makes the stomach dry. Zhuling Decoction （猪 苓 汤，polyporus decoction） promotes urination.

【英译】

Line 225

[The disease，characterized by] floating and slow pulse，external heat and internal cold，and diarrhea with undigested food，[can be] treated by Sini Decoction (四逆汤，decoction for resolving four kinds of adverseness).

【英译】

Line 226

If there is deficiency-cold in the stomach [and the patient is] unable to eat，drinking water will cause retch.

【原文】

(二二七)

脉浮,发热,口干,鼻燥,能食者则衄。

【今译】

脉浮发热,口干鼻燥,能进食的,就会发生鼻衄。

【原文】

(二二八)

阳明病,下之,其外有热,手足温,不结胸,心中懊憹,饥不能食,但头汗出者,栀子豉汤主之。

【今译】

阳明病,用泻下法治疗,身热未除,手足温热,无结胸表现,心中烦躁异常,虽感饥饿却不能进食,唯头部出汗的,可用栀子豉汤主治。

【原文】

(二二九)

阳明病,发潮热,大便溏,小便自可,胸胁满不去者,与小柴胡汤。

【今译】

阳明病,发潮热,大便溏薄,小便正常,但胸胁部闷满不解的,可以小柴胡汤治之。

Differentiation of pulse and syndrome/pattern [related to] yangming disease and treatment

【英译】

Line 227

[When there are symptoms and signs of] floating pulse, fever, dry mouth and dry nose, taking food will cause epistaxis.

【英译】

Line 228

[When] yangming disease [is treated by] purgation, [there are symptoms and signs of] external heat, warm hands and feet, anguish in the heart, hunger with difficulty to eat and sweating only over the head. Zhizi Chi Decoction (栀子豉汤, gardenia and fermented soybean decoction) [can be used] to treat it.

【英译】

Line 229

[In] yangming disease, there is tidal fever and sloppy stool, urination is normal but fullness is in the chest and rib-side is not resolved. [It] can be treated by Xiao Chaihu Decoction (小柴胡汤, minor bupleurium decoction).

【原文】

(二三〇)

阳明病,胁下鞕满,不大便而呕,舌上白苔者,可与小柴胡汤。上焦得通,津液得下,胃气因和,身濈然汗出而解。

【今译】

阳明病,胁下痞硬胀满,大便不解,呕吐,舌苔白,可用小柴胡汤治疗。用药后,上焦畅通,津液能够下达,胃气因此和顺,全身因而畅汗,疾病因之而解。

【原文】

(二三一)

阳明中风,脉弦浮大而短气,腹都满,胁下及心痛,久按之气不通,鼻干,不得汗,嗜卧,一身及目悉黄,小便难,有潮热,时时哕,耳前后肿,刺之小差,外不解。病过十日,脉续浮者,与小柴胡汤。

【今译】

阳明中风,脉象弦浮大,短气,全腹胀满,两胁及心下疼痛,按压很久但气仍然不畅通,鼻中干燥,无汗出,嗜睡,全身及目均发黄,小便困难,发潮热,干呕不断,耳前耳后肿胀。针刺治疗后病情稍减,但外症未解。病症发作十余天后,脉象依然弦浮的,可用小柴胡汤治疗。

Differentiation of pulse and syndrome/pattern [related to] yangming disease and treatment

【英译】

Line 230

[In] yangming disease, [if there are symptoms and signs of] stiffness and fullness below the rib-side, difficulty to defecate, vomiting and white tongue fur, Xiao Chaihu Decoction（小柴胡汤, minor bupleurium decoction） [can be used] to treat it. [After treatment,] the upper energizer will be able to unblock, fluid and humor will descend, stomach qi will be harmonized, and [there will be] general sweating. [As a result,] the disease will be cured.

【英译】

Line 231

Yangming [disease with] wind stroke [is characterized by] taut, floating and large pulse, shortness of breath, distension and fullness in the whole abdomen, pain below the rib-side and the heart, qi blockage under pressure for a long time, dryness of nose, absence of sweating, somnolence, yellowing of the whole body including the eyes, difficulty in urination, tidal fever, frequent retching and swelling in front of and behind the ears. [When treated by] acupuncture, [the disease is] slightly alleviated, [but] the external [syndrome/pattern] is not resolved. [If] the pulse is still floating [after] ten days [of occurrence], Xiao Chaihu Decoction（小柴胡汤, minor bupleurum decoction) [can be used] to treat it.

【原文】

(二三二)

脉但浮,无余证者,与麻黄汤。若不尿,腹满加哕者,不治。

【今译】

脉象若浮,而无其他症候,可用麻黄汤治疗。若无小便,但腹满与干呕更甚,属不治之症。

【原文】

(二三三)

阳明病,自汗出,若发汗,小便自利者,此为津液内竭,虽鞕不可攻之,当须自欲大便,宜蜜煎导而通之,若土瓜根及大猪胆汁,皆可为导。

蜜煎方

食蜜七合。

右一味,于铜器内微火煎,当须凝如饴状,搅之勿令焦着,欲可丸,并手捻作挺,令头锐,大如指,长两寸许,当热时急作,冷则硬,以内谷道中,以手急抱,欲大便时乃去之。(疑非仲景意,已试甚良)

又大猪胆一枚,泻汁,和少许醋,以灌谷道内,如一食顷,当大便出宿食恶物,甚效。

【今译】

阳明病,汗自出,若再行发汗,而小便又通畅的,则使体内津液枯竭,大便硬结,但不可攻泻。须待病人想解大便时,用蜜煎导引通便,或土瓜根及大猪胆汁,均可作为导药。

Differentiation of pulse and syndrome/pattern [related to] yangming disease and treatment

【英译】

Line 232

If the pulse is floating but there are no other syndromes/patterns, [it can be] treated by Mahuang Decoction (麻黄汤, ephedra decoction). If there is no urine but abdominal fullness and hiccup are more serious, [it is] fatal.

【英译】

Line 233

[In] yangming disease with spontaneous sweating, if perspiration is induced and urination is normal, it indicates internal exhaustion of fluid and humor. Although stool is hard, [it] cannot [be treated by] attack. [The doctor] should wait till the patient wants to defecate [and then] use Mijian Decoction (蜜煎方, boiled honey decoction) to promote defecation. [Besides,] Tuguagen (土瓜根, Japanese snakegourd root, Radix Trichosanthis Cucumeroidis) and a big pig bile can also be used to promote defecation.

Mijian Decoction (蜜煎方, boiled honey decoction) [is composed of] 7 *ge* of Shimi (食蜜, honey, Mel).

This ingredient is boiled in a copper pot with mild flame. It must be congealed like malt sugar, stirring repeatedly to avoid burning. To form [it into] pills, [one should] roll it with hands into a finger-shaped form with sharp tip, about two *cun* long. [It] should be used immediately when hot. [It will become] hard [when] cold. [When using the pill,] insert it into the anus, hold [the buttocks] tight with the hand and release [the buttocks] when about to defecate. (It is doubtful [whether this decoction] is Zhang Zhongjing's formula, [but it has] proved to be effective.)

A large pig bile [is selected] for promoting defecation. [It] is mixed with some vinegar and injected into the anus as enema. [It is] quiet effective in discharging undigested food and retained stool in defecation.

【原文】

(二三四)

阳明病,脉迟,汗出多,微恶寒者,表未解也。可发汗,宜桂枝汤。

【今译】

阳明病,脉象迟,汗出多,略微怕冷,是表症仍未解除,可发汗,适宜用桂枝汤主治。

【原文】

(二三五)

阳明病,脉浮,无汗而喘者,发汗则愈,宜麻黄汤。

【今译】

阳明病,脉象浮,无汗而又喘促,可用发汗法治愈,麻黄汤适合主治。

【原文】

(二三六)

阳明病,发热,汗出者,此为热越,不能发黄也。但头汗出,身无汗,剂颈而还,小便不利,渴引水浆者,此为瘀热在里,身必发黄,茵陈蒿汤

Differentiation of pulse and syndrome/pattern [related to] yangming disease and treatment

【英译】

Line 234

[In] yangming disease，slow pulse，profuse sweating and slight aversion to cold indicate that external [syndrome/pattern] is not resolved. [It can be treated by] diaphoresis with Guizhi Decoction (桂枝汤，cinnamon twig decoction).

【英译】

Line 235

Yangming disease，[characterized by] floating pulse，no sweating and panting，[can be] cured by diaphoresis. Mahuang Decoction（麻黄汤，ephedra decoction）is the appropriate [formula].

【英译】

Line 236

[In] yangming disease，fever and sweating indicate heat that has leaked out. [That is why] yellowishness（jaundice）will not be caused. But [if] sweating is just running from the head to the neck，not involving the body，urination is inhibited and [the patient] wants to drink water，it indicates internal stagnation of heat and the body must turn yellow. Yinchenhao Decoction（茵陈蒿汤，capillaris decoction）[can be used] to treat it.

Yinchenhao Decoction（茵陈蒿汤，capillaris decoction）[is

主之。

茵陈蒿汤方

茵陈蒿六两、栀子十四枚（擘）、大黄二两（去皮）。

右三味，以水一斗两升，先煮茵陈，减六升，内二味，煮取三升，去滓，分三服。小便当利，尿如皂角汁状，色正赤，一宿腹减，黄从小便去也。

【今译】

阳明病，发热汗出的，为热邪发越于外，所以不可形成黄症。如果仅头部出汗，到颈部为止，身上并无汗，小便不通畅，口渴想饮汤水，此为湿热郁滞在里，肌肤必然发黄。可以用茵陈蒿汤主治。

【原文】

（二三七）

阳明证，其人喜忘者，必有畜血，所以然者，本有久瘀血，故令喜忘，屎虽鞕，大便反易，其色必黑者，宜抵当汤下之。

【今译】

阳明病症中，有健忘症的病人，体内必有蓄血。原因在于瘀血久停，导致气血阻滞，因而使人健忘。大便虽然硬结，但反而易于解出，颜色一定为黑，可用抵当汤予以攻下。

Differentiation of pulse and syndrome / pattern [related to] yangming disease and treatment

composed of] 6 *liang* of Yinchenhao（茵陈蒿，capillaries，Herba Artemisia Capillaris），14 pieces of Zhizi（栀子，gardenia，Fructus Gardeniae）(break) and 2 *liang* of Dahuang（大黄，rhubarb，Radix et Rhizoma Rhei）(remove the bark).

These three ingredients are decocted in 1 *dou* and 2 *sheng* of water. Yinchenhao（茵陈蒿，capillaries，Herba Artemisia Capillaris）is decocted first to reduce 6 *sheng* [of water]. [Then] the other two ingredients are put into it [to boil] and get 3 *sheng*. The dregs are removed and [the decoction is] divided into three [doses] to take. [After taking the decoction,] urinination will be normalized and the urine appears like juice of gleditsia fruit，purely red in color. [After] one night，abdominal distension will be relieved and yellowishness（jaundice）will be discharged with urine.

【英译】

Line 237

[In] yangming syndrome/pattern，the patient with amnesia must have blood amassment. The reason is that there is blood stasis for a long time，therefore causing amnesia. Although the stool is hard，it is easy to defecate and the color is black. Didang Decoction （抵当汤，decoction for prevention）can be used to purge and attack it.

【原文】

(二三八)

阳明病,下之,心中懊侬而烦,胃中有燥屎者,可攻。腹微满,初头鞭,后必溏,不可攻之。若有燥屎者,宜大承气汤。

【今译】

阳明病,泻下后心中懊侬烦闷,肠胃中有燥屎的,可用攻下法。若腹部微有胀满,大便必先硬后溏,不可攻下。若有燥屎内结,可用大承气汤主治。

【原文】

(二三九)

病人不大便五六日,绕脐痛,烦躁,发作有时者,此有燥屎,故使不大便也。

【今译】

病人五六日期间未大便,环脐疼痛,烦躁不安,定时发作,因肠中有燥屎,所以大便不通畅。

Differentiation of pulse and syndrome / pattern [related to] yangming disease and treatment

【英译】

Line 238

[In] yangming disease, [after] purgation, [there are symptoms and signs of] anguish, vexation and dry stool in the [intestines and] stomach, [therapy for] attack can be used. [If there is] mild fullness in the abdomen and stool is first hard and then sloppy, [therapy for] attack cannot be used. If there is dry stool, Da Chengqi Decoction (大承气汤, major decoction for harmonizing qi) [can be used] to treat it.

【英译】

Line 239

The patient does not defecate for five to six days [with the symptoms and signs of] pain around the navel, vexation and periodic occurrence. There is dry stool in the intestines. That is why defecation is difficult.

【原文】

(二四〇)

病人烦热,汗出则解,又如疟状。日晡所发热者,属阳明也。脉实者,宜下之;脉浮虚者,宜发汗。下之,与大承气汤;发汗,宜桂枝汤。

【今译】

病人心中烦发热,汗出之后就能解除,但又像疟疾一样。午后定时发热,属于阳明里热。脉象实的,可以下法治之;脉象浮虚的,可以汗法治之。下法可用大承气汤,发汗可用桂枝汤。

【原文】

(二四一)

大下后,六七日不大便,烦不解,腹满痛者,此有燥屎也。所以然者,本有宿食故也,宜大承气汤。

【今译】

若以峻泻药攻下后,病人六七天不大便,烦躁不解,腹部胀满疼痛,此为肠中有燥屎所致。之所以如此,是因为本来有宿食的缘故,适宜用大承气汤治疗。

Differentiation of pulse and syndrome / pattern [related to] yangming disease and treatment

【英译】

Line 240

[If there is] vexing heat in the heart of the patient, [it will be] relieved after sweating, but appearing like malaria. [If] there is fever in the afternoon, [it] pertains to [internal heat in] yangming. [If] the pulse is in excess, purgation is appropriate; if the pulse is floating and weak, diaphoresis is appropriate. For purgation, Da Chengqi Decoction (大承气汤, major decoction for harmonizing qi) is appropriate; for diaphoresis, Guizhi Decoction (桂枝汤, cinnamon twig decoction) is appropriate.

【英译】

Line 241

After [application of] great purgation, the patient does not defecate for six or seven days, vexation is not relieved, [and there is still] abdominal fullness and pain, this is caused by dry stool [in the intestines]. The reason is that originally there is [accumulation of] undigested food. The appropriate [treatment is] Da Chengqi Decoction (大承气汤, major decoction for harmonizing qi).

【原文】

(二四二)

病人小便不利,大便乍难乍易,时有微热,喘冒不能卧者,有燥屎也。宜大承气汤。

【今译】

病人小便不利,大便时难时易,时有轻微发热,喘息,昏冒,不能安卧,此为燥屎阻结所致,宜用大承气汤治疗。

【原文】

(二四三)

食谷欲呕,属阳明也。吴茱萸汤主之。得汤反剧者,属上焦也。

吴茱萸汤方

吴茱萸一升(洗)、人参三两、生姜六两(切)、大枣十二枚(擘)。

右四味,以水七升,煮取二升,去滓,温服七合,日三服。

【今译】

病人食后想呕吐,属于阳明胃寒症,可用吴茱萸汤主治。如果服用吴茱萸汤后呕吐反而剧烈,则属上焦有热。

Differentiation of pulse and syndrome/pattern [related to] yangming disease and treatment

【英译】

Line 242

[When] the patient [suffers from] dysuria, now difficult and then easy, occasional slight sweating, panting, dizziness and difficulty to sleep, it is due to dry stool [in the intestines]. The appropriate [treatment is] Da Chengqi Decoction (大承气汤, major decoction for harmonizing qi).

【英译】

Line 243

[After] taking food, [the patient] feels nauseous, [it] is [stomach cold in] yangming [syndrome/pattern] and [can be] treated by Wuzhuyu Decoction (吴茱萸汤, evodia decoction). [If nausea is] severe after taking the decoction, [it] is due to [heat] in the upper energizer.

Wuzhuyu Decoction (吴茱萸汤, evodia decoction) [is composed of] 1 *sheng* of Wuzhuyu (吴茱萸, evodia, Fructus Evodiae) (wash), 3 *liang* of Renshen (人参, ginseng, Radix Ginseng), 6 liang of Shengjiang (生姜, fresh ginger, Rhizoma Zingberis Recens) (cut) and 12 pieces of Dazao (大枣, jujube, Fructus Ziziphus Jujubae) (break).

These four ingredients are decocted in 7 sheng of water to get 2 sheng. [After] removal of the dregs, [the decoction is] taken warm, 7 ge [each time] and three [times] a day.

【原文】

(二四四)

太阳病,寸缓,关浮,尺弱,其人发热汗出,复恶寒,不呕,但心下痞者,此以医下之也;如其不下者,病人不恶寒而渴者,此转属阳明也。小便数者,大便必鞕,不更衣十日,无所苦也。渴欲饮水,少少与之,但以法救之。渴者,宜五苓散。

【今译】

太阳病,寸脉缓,关脉浮,尺脉弱,病人发热,汗出,怕冷,不呕吐,心下痞满,此为医生误用攻下之法所致。如果没有攻下,病人出现不怕冷而口渴症状的,为邪传阳明所致。如果小便次数多,大便干硬,十余天不大便,但却没有痛苦之感。如果病人口渴想要喝水,可饮少量汤水,津液恢复了,病就可愈了。病人感到口渴的,宜用五苓散主治。

【原文】

(二四五)

脉阳微而汗出少者,为自和也。汗出多者,为太过。阳脉实,因发其汗,出多者,亦为太过。太过者,为阳绝于里,亡津液,大便因鞕也。

【今译】

阳脉微弱,汗出少的,属于自和。如果汗出多,则为太过。阳脉有力,是由于发汗而汗出太多,也属于太过。太过则阳气盛于里,导致阴液耗伤,大便因而干硬。

Differentiation of pulse and syndrome/pattern [related to] yangming disease and treatment

【英译】

Line 244

Taiyang disease, [characterized by] slow cun pulse, floating guan pulse, weak chi pulse, fever, sweating, aversion to cold without nausea and lump below the heart, is caused by [application of] purgation. If purgation is not used, the patient does not fear cold, but feels thirsty, it is due to [transmission of pathogenic factors to] yangming. [Although] urination is frequent, stool is not hard and [there is] no defecation for ten days, [the patient] does not feel uncomfortable. [If the patient] wants to drink water, give him small amount [of water]. Only [when such a] method [is used can the disease be] cured. [If the patient feels] thirsty, Wuling Powder (五苓散, wuling powder, made of five medicinal herbs) is appropriate [to treat it].

【英译】

Line 245

[When] yang pulse is lightly weak and sweating is scanty, [it] indicates spontaneous harmonization. [If] sweating is profuse, [it] is excess. [When] yang pulse is very strong, [it] is caused by diaphoresis. [If] sweating is profuse [after application of diaphoresis], [it] is also excess. Excess indicates exuberance of yang in the internal and exhaustion of fluid and humor, [consequently] resulting in hard stool.

【原文】

(二四六)

脉浮而芤,浮为阳,芤为阴,浮芤相搏,胃气生热,其阳则绝。

【今译】

脉浮而芤,浮为阳气盛,芤为阴血虚,浮脉与芤脉相搏,导致胃气生热,阳热亢盛至极。

【原文】

(二四七)

趺阳脉浮而涩,浮则胃气强,涩则小便数,浮涩相搏,大便则鞭,其脾为约,麻子仁丸主之。

麻子仁丸方

麻子仁两升、芍药半斤、枳实半斤(炙)、大黄一斤(去皮)、厚朴一尺(炙,去皮)、杏仁一升(去皮尖,熬,别作脂)。

右六味,蜜和丸,如梧桐子大,饮服十丸,日三服,渐加,以知为度。

【今译】

趺阳脉浮涩,浮因胃热盛,涩因小便数,浮脉与涩脉同时相搏,大便则硬,为脾被胃热约束所致,可用麻子仁丸主治。

Differentiation of pulse and syndrome/pattern [related to] yangming disease and treatment

【英译】

Line 246

The pulse is floating and [hollow like] scallion-stalk. Floating [pulse] indicates [exuberance of] yang while [hollow pulse like] scallion-stalk indicates [deficiency of] yin [blood]. Conflict of floating [pulse] and [hollow pulse like] scallion-stalk produces heat in stomach qi, enabling yang to prevail to the extreme.

【英译】

Line 247

Fuyang pulse (located in the upper suface of the foot on the stomach meridian of foot-yangming) is floating and rough. Floating [pulse] indicates that stomach qi is strong while rough [pulse] indicates frequent urination. Conflict of the floating [pulse] and rough [pulse] indicates hard stool caused by restriction of the spleen. [It can be] treated by Maziren Pill (麻子仁丸, hemp seed pill).

Maziren Pill (麻子仁丸, hemp seed pill) [is composed of] 2 *sheng* of Maziren (麻子仁, hemp seed, Semen Cannbis), 0.5 *jin* of Shaoyao (芍药, peony, Radix Paeoniae), 0.5 *jin* of Zhishi (枳实, processed unripe bitter orange, Fructus Aurantii Immaturus) (broil), 1 *jin* of Dahuang (大黄, rhubarb, Radix et Rhizoma Rhei) (remove the bark), 1 *chi* of Houpo (厚朴, magnolia bark, Cortex Magnoliae Officinalis) (broil and remove the bark) and 1 *jin* of Xingren (杏仁, apricot kernel, Semen Armeniacae Amarum) (remove peel and tips, simmer, grind into the form like fat).

These six ingredients are mixed with honey to produce pills like firmiana seeds. Take ten pills with water [each time] and three times a day. [The dose can] gradually increase till effective.

【原文】

(二四八)

太阳病三日,发汗不解,蒸蒸发热者,属胃也,调胃承气汤主之。

【今译】

太阳病,三天之后,以发汗法治疗而不解,高热炽盛的,表明其已转属于胃,可用调胃承气汤主治。

【原文】

(二四九)

伤寒吐后,腹胀满者,与调胃承气汤。

【今译】

伤寒,用吐法治疗之后,腹部胀满的,可以调胃承气汤主治。

【原文】

(二五〇)

太阳病,若吐、若下、若发汗后,微烦,小便数,大便因鞭者,与小承气汤,和之愈。

【今译】

太阳病,如果用催吐、攻下或发汗法治疗后,出现轻微心烦、小便频数、大便硬结,可用小承气汤治疗,和畅而痊愈。

Differentiation of pulse and syndrome／pattern ［related to］ yangming disease and treatment

【英译】

Line 248

Taiyang disease，three days ［after occurrence］，is not resolved ［after application of］ diaphoresis and there is profuse sweating，indicating ［that the disease is already］ transmitted to the stomach. ［It can be］ treated by Tiaowei Chengqi Decoction（调胃承气汤，decoction for regulating the stomach and harmonizing qi）.

【英译】

Line 249

［In］ cold damage，after ［treatment with］ vomiting ［therapy］，there is abdominal distension and fullness. ［It should be］ treated by Tiaowei Chengqi Decoction（调胃承气汤，decoction for regulating the stomach and harmonizing qi）.

【英译】

Line 250

［In］ taiyang disease，if ［treated by therapeutic methods for］ vomiting，purgation and diaphoresis，［there are still symptoms and signs of］ slight vexation，frequent urination and hard stool，［it should be］ treated by Xiao Chengqi Decoction（小承气汤，minor decoction for harmonizing qi）to harmonize ［stomach qi］ and cure ［the disease］.

【原文】

(二五一)

得病二三日,脉弱,无太阳、柴胡证,烦躁,心下鞕,至四五日,虽能食,以小承气汤少少与,微和之,令小安。至六日,与承气汤一升。若不大便六七日,小便少者,虽不受食,但初头硬,后必溏,未定成鞕,攻之必溏,须小便利,屎定鞕,乃可攻之,宜大承气汤。

【今译】

患者得病两三天,脉弱,没有太阳证和柴胡证,烦躁不安,胃脘胀硬。到了四五天,虽然能进食,可用小承气汤治疗,但只能用量小以和胃气,使病人略感安宁。到了第六天,再令其服小承气汤一升。如果六七日后仍然不大便,小便也少,虽然不能进食,也不可攻下,因为仅是初期大便硬,之后则溏薄,并非完全燥硬。误用攻下,大便必然只燥硬而不溏薄。只有小便通利,大便开始燥硬的时候,才可攻下。可用大承气汤主治。

Differentiation of pulse and syndrome/pattern [related to] yangming disease and treatment

【英译】

Line 251

Two or three days [after occurrence of] disease, the pulse is weak, there are no taiyang [syndrome/pattern] and Chaihu [Decoction (柴胡汤, bupleurum decoction) syndrome/pattern], [and there are] vexation and lump below the heart. Four or five days later, [the patient is] able to eat, Xiao Chengqi Decoction (小承气汤, minor decoction for harmonizing qi) [can be used to treat it], [but the amount should be] small so as to harmonize [stomach] and tranquilize [the patient]. Six days later, [the patient should take] 1 *sheng* of [Xiao] Chengqi Decoction (小承气汤, minor decoction for harmonizing qi). If there is no defecation in six or seven days [after occurrence] and urine is scanty, though [the patient will] not take food, [the fact is that] stool at the beginning is hard and then sloppy, not always hard. [If] purgation [therapy is used,] sloppy [stool will inevitably become] hard. Only when urination is normal and stool is hard can purgation [therapy be used]. The appropriate [therapy is] Da Chengqi Decoction (大承气汤, major decoction for harmonizing qi).

【原文】

(二五二)

伤寒六七日,目中不了了,睛不和,无表里证,大便难,身微热者,此为实也。急下之,宜大承气汤。

【今译】

伤寒发作六七天后,患者视物不清,眼球转动不灵,没有表里之证,大便不畅,轻微发热。这是燥热内结而成的实证,应采用急下之法,适宜用以急下的是大承气汤。

【原文】

(二五三)

阳明病,发热、汗多者,急下之,宜大承气汤。

【今译】

阳明病,有发热、汗多等症状的,可采用急下之法。适宜用以急下的是大承气汤。

Differentiation of pulse and syndrome / pattern [related to] yangming disease and treatment

【英译】

Line 252

Six or seven days [after occurrence of] cold damage, [there are symptoms and signs of] unclear vision, dullness of the eyes, no external or internal syndrome/pattern, difficulty in defecation and slight fever. [It should be treated by] drastic purgation. The appropriate [formula] is Da Chengqi Decoction (大承气汤, major decoction for harmonizing qi).

【英译】

Line 253

[In] yangming disease, [if there are symptoms and signs of] fever and profuse sweating, [it should be treated by] drastic purgation. The appropriate [formula] is Da Chengqi Decoction (大承气汤, major decoction for harmonizing qi).

【原文】

(二五四)

发汗不解,腹满痛者,急下之,宜大承气汤。

【今译】

发汗之后病未解除,但却出现腹部胀满疼痛等症状的,可采用急下之法。适宜用以急下的是大承气汤。

【原文】

(二五五)

腹满不减,减不足言,当下之,宜大承气汤。

【今译】

腹部胀满,始终未减,即使偶尔略有轻减,也微不足道,可采用下法治之。适宜用的是大承气汤。

Differentiation of pulse and syndrome / pattern [related to] yangming disease and treatment

【英译】

Line 254

[After application of] diaphoresis，the disease is not resolved，[and there is] abdominal fullness and pain. [It should be treated by] drastic purgation. The appropriate [formula] is Da Chengqi Decoction (大承气汤，major decoction for harmonizing qi).

【英译】

Line 255

Abdominal distension and fullness are not reduced. [Even if occasionally] reduced some，[it is still] not worth mentioning. [It should be treated by] purgation. The appropriate [formula] is Da Chengqi Decoction (大承气汤，major decoction for harmonizing qi).

【原文】

(二五六)

阳明、少阳合病，必下利，其脉不负者，为顺也。负者，失也。互相克贼，名为负也。脉滑而数者，有宿食也，当下之，宜大承气汤。

【今译】

阳明、少阳两经合病，必然发生腹泻。如果脉象不偏，为顺症；脉象若偏，则为逆症。相互克制的，即为逆相。脉象滑而数，说明有宿食内停，应当以攻下治之，可用大承气汤。

【原文】

(二五七)

病人无表里证，发热七八日，虽脉浮数者，可下之。假令已下，脉数不解，合热则消谷喜饥，至六七日，不大便者，有瘀血，宜抵当汤。

【今译】

病人没有表证和里证，发热已经七八天了，虽然脉象浮数，但也可以用下法。如果使用泻下法治疗后，脉数不变，热合于血分则消谷善饥。六七日后不大便的，是因为有瘀血内结，宜用抵当汤治疗。

Differentiation of pulse and syndrome / pattern [related to] yangming disease and treatment

【英译】

Line 256

Disease involving both yangming and shaoyang [meridians] will cause diarrhea. [If] the pulse is not adverse, it is favourable; [if the pulse is] adverse, [it is] deviation. [If there is] mutual restriction, [it is known as] adverse. [If] the pulse is slippery and rapid, [it indicates] indigestion. [It should be treated by] purgation. The appropriate [formula] is Da Chengqi Decoction (大承气汤, major decoction for harmonizing qi).

【英译】

Line 257

The patient does not have external or internal syndrome/ pattern, there is fever for seven or eight days. Although the pulse is floating and rapid, purgation can [be used to treat] it. If purgation is already used, [but] the pulse is not changed and heat has combined [with the blood], [there will be] swift digestion and frequent hunger. Six or seven days [after occurrence, if there is] no defecation, [it indicates that] there is blood stasis. The appropriate [treatment] is Didang Decoction (抵当汤, prevention decoction).

【原文】

(二五八)

若脉数不解,而下不止,必协热便脓血也。

【今译】

攻下之后如果脉数不解,而且又腹泻不止,必然出现协热下利、解脓便血的变症。

【原文】

(二五九)

伤寒发汗已,身目为黄,所以然者,以寒湿在里不解故也。以为不可下也,于寒湿中求之。

【今译】

伤寒发汗以后,皮肤与眼睛皆发黄,之所以出现这种症状,是因为寒湿在里未能解除。治疗发黄不可以用下法,应采用治疗寒湿之法。

Differentiation of pulse and syndrome/pattern [related to] yangming disease and treatment

【英译】

Line 258

[After application of purgation, if] the pulse is not changed and [there is] still frequent diarrhea, there must be complex diarrhea with bloody pus.

【英译】

Line 259

[In] cold damage, after [application of] diaphoresis, the skin and eyes become yellow. The reason is that cold dampness in the internal is not resolved. It is obvious that purgation should not be used and [the treatment can only be] selected [from those used to treat] cold dampness.

【原文】

(二六〇)

伤寒七八日,身黄如橘子色,小便不利,腹微满者,茵蔯蒿汤主之。

【今译】

伤寒六七天后,皮肤发黄,状如橘子之色,小便不通畅,腹部稍感胀满,可用茵陈蒿汤主治。

【原文】

(二六一)

伤寒,身黄,发热者,栀子柏皮汤主之。

栀子柏皮汤方

肥栀子十五个(擘)、甘草一两(炙)、黄柏二两。

右三味,以水四升,煮取一升半,去滓,分温再服。

【今译】

伤寒,周身发黄,且发热的,可用栀子柏皮汤治疗。

Differentiation of pulse and syndrome / pattern [related to] yangming disease and treatment

【英译】

Line 260

Six or seven days [after occurrence of] cold damage [disease], the whole skin becomes as yellow as tangerine, urination is inhibited and [there is] slight abdominal fullness. Yinchenhao Decoction (茵陈蒿汤, capillaries decoction) [can be used] to treat it.

【英译】

Line 261

[In] cold damage [disease], [if] the whole body is yellow and there is fever, Zhizi Baipi Decoction (栀子柏皮汤, gardenia and phellodendron decoction) [can be used] to treat it.

Zhizi Baipi Decoction (栀子柏皮汤, gardenia and phellodendron decoction) [is composed of] 15 pieces of fat Zhizi (栀子, gardenia, Fructus Gardeniae) (break), 1 *liang* of Gancao (甘草, licorice, Radix Glycyrrhizae Praeparata) (broil) and 2 *liang* of Huangbo (黄柏, phellodendron, Cortex Phellodendri).

These three ingredients are decocted in 4 *sheng* of water to get 1.5 *sheng* [after boiling]. [After] removal of the dregs, [the decoction is] divided [into two doses] and taken warm twice [a day].

【原文】

(二六二)

伤寒,瘀热在里,身必黄,麻黄连翘赤小豆汤主之。

麻黄连翘赤小豆汤方

麻黄二两(去节)、连翘二两(连翘根也)、杏仁四十个(去皮尖)、赤小豆一升、大枣十二枚(擘)、生梓白皮(切)一升、生姜二两(切)、甘草二两(炙)。

右八味,以潦水一斗,先煮麻黄再沸,去上沫,内诸药,煮取三升,去滓,分温三服,半日服尽。

【今译】

伤寒病中,如果有湿热郁滞在里,身体必定发黄,宜用麻黄连翘赤小豆汤主治。

Differentiation of pulse and syndrome/pattern [related to] yangming disease and treatment

【英译】

Line 262

[In] cold damage [disease], [if there is] stagnated heat in the internal, the body will become yellow. [It should be] treated by Mahuang Lianqiao Chixiaodou Decoction (麻黄连翘赤小豆汤, ephedra, forsythia and rice bean decoction).

Mahuang Lianqiao Chixiaodou Decoction (麻黄连翘赤小豆汤, ephedra, forsythia and rice bean decoction) [is composed of] 2 *liang* of Mahuang (麻黄, ephedra, Herba Ephedrae) (remove the nodes), 2 *liang* of Lianqiao (连翘, forsythia root, Fructus Forsythiae), 40 pieces of Xingren (杏仁, apricot kernel, Semen Armeniacae Amarum) (remove the peel and tips), 1 *sheng* of Chixiaodou (赤小豆, rice bean, Vigna umbellata), 12 pieces of Dazao (大枣, jujube, Fructus Ziziphus Jujubae) (break), 1 *sheng* of raw Zibaipi (梓白皮, catalpa bark, Cortex Catalpae) (cut), 2 *liang* of Shengjiang (生姜, fresh ginger, Rhizoma Zingiberis Recens) (cut) and 2 *liang* of Gancao (甘草, licorice, Radix Glycyrrhizae Praeparata) (broil).

These eight ingredients are decocted in 1 *dou* of water. Mahuang (麻黄, ephedra, Herba Ephedrae) is boiled first. [Then it is] boiled again. [After] the foam is removed, other ingredients are put into it and boiled to get 3 *sheng*. [After] removal of dregs, [the decoction is] divided into three [doses] and taken warm three times. The whole [decoction is] taken in half a day.

辨少阳病脉证并治

【原文】

(二六三)

少阳之为病,口苦,咽干,目眩也。

【今译】

少阳病的症候,主要是口苦、咽喉干燥、头晕目眩。

【原文】

(二六四)

少阳中风,两耳无所闻,目赤,胸中满而烦者,不可吐下,吐下则悸而惊。

【今译】

少阳中风后,两耳无听力,眼睛发红,胸中满闷,烦扰不宁,不可用吐法和下法治疗。如果用吐下法治疗,会引起心悸和惊惕。

Differentiation of pulse and syndrome/pattern
[related to] shaoyang disease and treatment

Differentiation of pulse and syndrome/pattern [related to] shaoyang disease and treatment

【英译】

Line 263

[The major symptoms and signs of] shaoyang disease include bitterness in the mouth, dryness of the throat and dizziness.

【英译】

Line 264

Shaoyang [disease with] wind stroke [is characterized by] inability of both ears to listen, redness of the eyes, fullness in the chest and vexation. [It] cannot [be treated by therapeutic methods for] vomiting and purgation. Vomiting and purgation [treatment will] cause palpitation and fright.

【原文】

（二六五）

伤寒，脉弦细，头痛发热者，属少阳。少阳不可发汗，发汗则谵语，此属胃，胃和则愈；胃不和，烦而悸。

【今译】

伤寒病，脉象弦细，头痛发热，属少阳病。少阳病不可用发汗法治疗，误用发汗法会导致谵语，原因是津液受损，津伤胃燥。如果通过治疗使胃气得以调和，病就会痊愈。如果胃气不和，就会出现烦躁、心悸。

【原文】

（二六六）

本太阳病不解，转入少阳者，胁下鞕满，干呕不能食，往来寒热，尚未吐下，脉沉紧者，与小柴胡汤。

【今译】

原本患太阳病，但却未予解除，使得病邪传入少阳，导致胁下痞硬胀满，干呕，不能进食，寒热交替发作。如果没有使用涌吐或攻下法而脉象沉紧的，可用小柴胡汤治疗。

Differentiation of pulse and syndrome/pattern [related to] shaoyang disease and treatment

【英译】

Line 265

[In] cold damage [disease], [if] the pulse is taut and thin, and [there is] headache with fever, [it] is shaoyang syndrome/pattern. Shaoyang [disease] cannot [be treated by] diaphoresis. [Wrong use of] diaphoresis will cause delirium due to [injury of] the stomach [by exhaustion of fluid and humor]. [If] the stomach is harmonized, [the disease will be] cured. [If] the stomach is not harmonized, vexation and palpitation [will be caused].

【英译】

Line 266

[If] the original taiyang disease is not resolved, [the pathogenic factors will] transmit to shaoyang [meridian], [consequently causing] hardness and fullness below the rib-side, dry retching, inability to take food, alternation of cold and heat and sunken and tight pulse. [It can be] treated by Xiao Chaihu Decoction (小柴胡汤, minor bupleurum decoction).

【原文】

(二六七)

若已吐下发汗温针,谵语,柴胡汤证罢,此为坏病,知犯何逆,以法治之。

【今译】

如果已用过催吐、泻下、发汗、温针等方法治疗,病人依然有谵语之症,而柴胡汤证并不存在,这已成为恶性疾病。应谨慎检查其属于何种误法所致,应用适宜之法治疗。

【原文】

(二六八)

三阳合病,脉浮大,上关上,但欲眠睡,目合则汗。

【今译】

太阳、阳明、少阳三经合病,脉象浮大,弦直于关部,只想睡眠,闭眼则出汗。

Differentiation of pulse and syndrome/pattern [related to] shaoyang disease and treatment

【英译】

Line 267

If ［the therapeutic methods for］ promoting vomiting, purgation and sweating ［as well as acupuncture with］ warmed needle are used, ［there is still］ delirium, ［but there is］ no ［Xiao］ Chaihu ［Decoction］（小柴胡汤, minor bupleurum decoction）syndrome/pattern. This is a fatal disease. ［The doctor must be］ aware ［that it is caused by］ wrong ［treatment］ and ［try to find appropriate］ method to treat it.

【英译】

Line 268

［When］ the disease involving three yang（taiyang, yangming and shaoyang）, the pulse is floating, large and ［extending］ upwards to the guan ［region］, ［the patient］ only wants to sleep, but ［when closing］ the eyes ［there will be］ sweating.

【原文】

（二六九）

伤寒六七日，无大热，其人躁烦者，此为阳去入阴故也。

【今译】

伤寒病发作六七日后，身体没有大热，但病人却烦躁不安，这是外邪入里所致。

【原文】

（二七〇）

伤寒三日，三阳为尽，三阴当受邪，其人反能食而不呕，此为三阴不受邪也。

【今译】

伤寒发作的第三天，邪已传尽三阳经，也应传入三阴经。若病人此时能够饮食而不呕吐，说明邪气并未传入三阴经。

Differentiation of pulse and syndrome/pattern [related to] shaoyang disease and treatment

【英译】

Line 269

Six or seven days [after occurrence of] cold damage [disease], there is no severe fever, [but] the patient feels vexing and restless. This is caused by external pathogenic factors entering the internal.

【英译】

Line 270

Three days [after occurrence of] cold damage [disease], [pathogenic factors have already] transmitted to the three yang [meridians] and also three yin [meridians]. [If] the patient is able to eat and does not vomit, it indicates that pathogenic factors have not transmitted to the three yin [meridians].

【原文】

(二七一)

伤寒三日,少阳脉小者,欲已也。

【今译】

伤寒发作三日后,病在少阳,脉象微小的,表明病将痊愈。

【原文】

(二七二)

少阳病欲解时,从寅至辰上。

【今译】

少阳病将解除的时间,一般从寅时(凌晨 3 点到 5 点)至辰时(上午 7 点到 9 点)之间。

Differentiation of pulse and syndrome / pattern [related to] shaoyang disease and treatment

【英译】

Line 271

Three days [after occurrence of] cold damage [disease], [the disease is transmitted to] shaoyang [meridian] and the pulse is tiny, [indicating that the disease is] about to heal.

【英译】

Line 272

[The time for] shaoyang disease to resolve is about from yin (3:00 − 5:00) to chen (7:00 − 9:00).

辨太阴病脉证并治

【原文】

(二七三)

太阴之为病,腹满而吐,食不下,自利益甚,时腹自痛。若下之,必胸下结鞕。

【今译】

太阴病的主要症候是,腹部胀满,呕吐,不能用餐,腹泻严重,腹部时时疼痛。若误用攻下法治疗,则会引起胃脘部硬结。

【原文】

(二七四)

太阴中风,四肢烦疼,脉阳微阴涩而长者,为欲愈。

【今译】

太阴中风,四肢烦疼痛,脉象由微涩而变长,是将痊愈的表现。

Differentiation of pulse and syndrome / pattern
[related to] taiyin disease and treatment

Differentiation of pulse and syndrome/pattern [related to] taiyin disease and treatment

【英译】

Line 273

Taiyin disease [is mainly characterized by] abdominal fullness, vomiting, inability to eat, severe diarrhea and frequent abdominal pain. If purgation [is used to treat] it, [it] will cause hardness and lump below the chest.

【英译】

Line 274

[In] taiyin [disease with] wind stroke, [there is] vexing pain in the four limbs and the slightly rough pulse becomes long, indicating [that the disease is] about to heal.

【原文】

(二七五)

太阴病,欲解时,从亥至丑上。

【今译】

太阴病将解除的时间,大致是在亥时(晚上 9—11 点)至丑时(凌晨 1—3 点)。

【原文】

(二七六)

太阴病,脉浮者,可发汗,宜桂枝汤。

【今译】

太阴病,如果脉浮,可以用汗法治疗,宜用桂枝汤。

【原文】

(二七七)

自利不渴者,属太阴,以其脏有寒故也。当温之,宜服四逆辈。

【今译】

腹泻而口不渴的,属太阴病,因脾脏虚寒所致,应以温里法治疗,宜服用四逆汤之类的方药。

Differentiation of pulse and syndrome/pattern [related to] taiyin disease and treatment

【英译】

Line 275

[The time for] taiyin disease to resolve is about from hai (21:00 - 23:00) to chou (1:00 - 3:00). `

【英译】

Line 276

[In] taiyin disease [if there is] pulse floating, [it] can [be treated by] diaphoresis. The appropriate [formula is] Guizhi Decoction (桂枝汤, cinnamon twig decoction).

【英译】

Line 277

Diarrhea without thirst belongs to taiyin disease due to cold in the spleen. Warming [therapy] can [be used to treat] it. Sini [Decoction] (四逆汤, decoction for resolving four kinds of adverseness) is [one of] the appropriate [kinds of formulas].

【原文】

(二七八)

伤寒,脉浮而缓,手足自温者,系在太阴。太阴当发身黄,若小便自利者,不能发黄,至七八日,虽暴烦下利,日十余行,必自止,以脾家实,腐秽当去故也。

【今译】

伤寒病,脉象浮缓,手足自然温暖的,病属太阴。病在太阴,患者应身发黄,若小便通畅,则不会形成黄症。七八天后,患者突然出现心烦,腹泻一天十多次,一定会自行停止。这是脾阳恢复后,腐秽之物随之祛除的缘故。

【原文】

(二七九)

本太阳病,医反下之,因尔腹满时痛者,属太阴也,桂枝加芍药汤主之。大实痛者,桂枝加大黄汤主之。

桂枝加芍药汤方

桂枝三两(去皮)、芍药六两、甘草二两(炙)、大枣十二枚(擘)、生姜三两(切)。

右五味,以水七升,煮取三升,去滓,温分三服。

本云桂枝汤,今加芍药。

Differentiation of pulse and syndrome/pattern [related to] taiyin disease and treatment

【英译】

Line 278

[In] cold damage，[there is] floating and slow pulse，the hands and feet are naturally warm，[indicating that the disease] is in taiyin. [When the disease] is in taiyin，[the patient's] body will become yellow. If urination is normal，[there will be] no yellow [syndrome/pattern]. Seven or eight days [after occurrence]，although there is severe vexing and diarrhea that occurs over ten times a day，[it will] certainly cease because the spleen is strong and can eliminate decayed and putrid [substance].

【英译】

Line 279

Originally [it is] taiyang disease. [When] treated by purgation，[it] causes abdominal fullness and frequent pain，indicating [that pathogenic factors have already entered] taiyin [meridian]. Guizhi Decoctiion（桂枝汤，cinnamon twig decoction）added with Shaoyao（芍药，peony，Radix Paeoniae）[can be used] to treat it. [If there is] great excessive pain，Guizhi Decoction（桂枝汤，cinnamon twig decoction）added with Dahuang（大黄，rhubarb，Radix et Rhizoma Rhei）[can be used] to treat it.

Guizhi Decoction（桂枝汤，cinnamon twig decoction）added with Shaoyao（芍药，peony，Radix Paeoniae）[is composed of] 3 *liang* of Guizhi（桂枝，cinnamon twig，Radix Glycyrrhizae Praeparata）（remove the bark），6 *liang* of（芍药，peony，Radix Paeoniae），2 *liang* of Gancao（甘草，licorice，Ramulus

桂枝加大黄汤方

桂枝三两（去皮）、大黄二两、芍药六两、生姜三两、甘草二两（炙）、大枣十二枚（擘）。

右六味，以水七升，煮取三升，去滓，温服一升，日三服。

【今译】

本为太阳病，医生反而用攻下法治之，引起腹中胀满，时时腹痛。这是邪陷太阴所致，宜用桂枝加芍药汤治疗。如有大实痛的，可用桂枝加大黄汤治疗。

【原文】

（二八〇）

太阴为病，脉弱，其人续自便利，设当行大黄、芍药者，宜减之，以其人胃气弱，易动故也。

【今译】

太阴病，脉象弱，病人暂时大便通利。应用大黄、芍药治疗此类患者时，应当减量使用。因为这类患者胃气虚弱，易受损伤。

Differentiation of pulse and syndrome / pattern [related to] taiyin disease and treatment

Cinnamomi) (broil), 12 pieces of Dazao (大枣, jujube, Fructus Ziziphus Jujubae) (break) and 3 *liang* of Shengjiang (生姜, fresh ginger, Radix Zingiberis Recens) (cut).

These five ingredients are decocted in 7 *sheng* of water to get 3 *sheng* [after] boiling. The dregs are removed and [the decoction is] divided [into three doses] and taken warm.

Guizhi Decoction (桂枝汤, cinnamon twig decoction) added with Dahuang (大黄, rhubarb, Radix et Rhizoma Rhei) [is composed of] 3 *liang* of Guizhi (桂枝, cinnamon twig, Radix Glycyrrhizae Praeparata) (remove the bark), 2 *liang* of Dahuang (大黄, rhubarb, Radix et Rhizoma Rhei), 6 *liang* of Shaoyao (芍药, peony, Radix Paeoniae), 3 *liang* of Shengjiang (生姜, fresh ginger, Radix Zingiberis Recens), 2 *liang* of Gancao (甘草, licorice, Ramulus Cinnamomi) (broil) and 12 pieces of Dazao (大枣, jujube, Fructus Ziziphus Jujubae) (break).

These six ingredients are decocted in 7 *sheng* of water to get 3 *sheng* [after] boiling. The dregs are removed and [the decoction is] taken 1 *sheng* warm [each time] and three times a day.

【英译】

Line 280

[In] taiyin disease, the pulse is weak and the patient temporarily defecates normally. To treat [such a patient] with Dahuang (大黄, rhubarb, Radix et Rhizoma Rhei) and Shaoyao (芍药, peony, Radix Paeoniae), [the dosage should be] reduced because stomach qi in the patient is weak and easy to be injured.

辨少阴病脉证并治

【原文】

(二八一)

少阴之为病,脉微细,但欲寐也。

【今译】

少阴病的症候,为脉象微细,病人昏昏沉沉欲睡。

【原文】

(二八二)

少阴病,欲吐不吐,心烦,但欲寐,五六日自利而渴者,属少阴也。虚故引水自救。若小便色白者,少阴病形悉具。小便白者,以下焦虚有寒,不能制水,故令色白也。

【今译】

少阴病中,患者想吐又不能吐,心里烦闷,昏昏欲睡。到了第五六日,腹泻而口渴的,属于少阴病症,口渴是由于津液不足而想通过引水以自救。如果小便色白,则少阴病的症候就完全具备了。小便之所以色白,是因为下焦有虚寒,不能制水,所以使小便颜色清白。

Differentiation of pulse and syndrome/pattern
[related to] shaoyin disease and treatment

Differentiation of pulse and syndrome/pattern [related to] shaoyin disease and treatment

【英译】

Line 281

Shaoyin disease [is characterized by] faint and feeble pulse and sleepiness.

【英译】

Line 282

[In] shaoyin disease, [the patient is] nauseous but cannot vomit, feeling vexing and sleepy. Five or six days [after occurrence, there is] diarrhea and thirst, belonging to shaoyin [disease]. [The patient feels thirsty and wants] to drink water [because fluid is] deficient. [So drinking water can] rescue himself. If urine is clear, all [the symptoms and signs of] shaoyin disease are present. [The reason why] urine is clear is that there is deficiency-cold in the lower energizer, failing to control water and therefore making [urine] clear.

【原文】

(二八三)

病人脉阴阳俱紧,反汗出者,亡阳也。此属少阴,法当咽痛而复吐利。

【今译】

病人尺寸部脉象均沉紧,本应无汗,但却出汗,这是亡阳的征象,属于少阴病,理应有呕吐、腹泻、咽喉疼痛等症状。

【原文】

(二八四)

少阴病,咳而下利,谵语者,被火气劫故也。小便必难,以强责少阴汗也。

【今译】

少阴病患者,有咳嗽、腹泻、谵语等症状,是误用火法所致。强发少阴汗,必然导致小便艰涩难下。

【原文】

(二八五)

少阴病,脉细沉数,病为在里,不可发汗。

【今译】

少阴病,脉象沉细数,为病在里,不宜用发汗法治疗。

Differentiation of pulse and syndrome/pattern [related to] shaoyin disease and treatment

【英译】

Line 283

Both yin and yang pulses of the patient are tight, and there is sweating, [indicating] loss of yang. [Such a case] belongs to shaoyin [disease] and there should be [the symptoms and signs of] sore-throat, vomiting and diarrhea.

【英译】

Line 284

[In] shaoyin disease, [there are symptoms and signs of] cough, diarrhea and delirium caused by [wrong use of] attacking [therapy] with fire qi. [As a result,] urination is inevitably difficult because sweating is forced in shaoyin [disease].

【英译】

Line 285

[In] shaoyin disease, the pulse is thin, sunken and rapid, [indicating that] the disease is in the internal and cannot [be treated by] diaphoresis.

【原文】

(二八六)

少阴病,脉微,不可发汗,亡阳故也。阳已虚,尺脉弱涩者,复不可下之。

【今译】

少阴病,脉象微,不可用发汗法治疗,是亡阳所致。阳已虚,尺脉又弱涩,也不可用泻下法治疗。

【原文】

(二八七)

少阴病,脉紧,至七八日,自下利,脉暴微,手足反温,脉紧反去者,为欲解也,虽烦,下利必自愈。

【今译】

少阴病患者,脉象紧。八九日后,腹泻,脉象突然微弱,手足反而发热,脉象不再紧,说明病患将解除。虽然患者依然有烦躁和腹泻的症状,但必然将会自愈。

Differentiation of pulse and syndrome／pattern ⌊related to⌋ shaoyin disease and treatment

【英译】

Line 286

⌊In⌋ shaoyin disease，the pulse is faint．⌊It⌋ cannot ⌊be treated by⌋ diaphoresis ⌊because it is caused by⌋ loss of yang．⌊When⌋ yang is deficient，chi pulse ⌊will be⌋ weak and rough，and purgation cannot ⌊be used to treat⌋ it.

【英译】

Line 287

⌊In⌋ shaoyin disease，the pulse is tight．Eight or nine days ⌊after occurrence，there is⌋ diarrhea，the pulse suddenly ⌊becomes⌋ faint，the hands and feet are warm，and the pulse is no longer tight. ⌊Such changes⌋ indicate ⌊that the disease is⌋ about to heal． Although there is still vexation and diarrhea，⌊the patient will⌋ spontaneously recover.

【原文】

(二八八)

少阴病,下利。若利自止,恶寒而蜷卧,手足温者,可治。

【今译】

少阴病患者,有腹泻之症。如果腹泻自行停止,患者恶寒,蜷卧在床,手足温热,还是可以治愈的。

【原文】

(二八九)

少阴病,恶寒而蜷,时自烦,欲去衣被者,可治。

【今译】

少阴病患者,恶寒而蜷卧,时时有烦躁之感,想脱掉衣揭开被子,其病还是可治的。

【原文】

(二九〇)

少阴中风,脉阳微阴浮者,为欲愈。

【今译】

少阴中风,阳脉微弱,阴脉虚浮,病情将要痊愈。

Differentiation of pulse and syndrome / pattern [related to] shaoyin disease and treatment

【英译】

Line 288

[In] shaoyin disease, [there is] diarrhea. If diarrhea ceases spontaneously, [the patient] aversion to cold, curls himself up to lie in bed with warm hands and feet, [the disease] can be cured.

【英译】

Line 289

[In] shaoyin disease, [the patient] aversion to cold, curls himself up to lie in bed with frequent vexation and desire to remove clothes and quilt. [The disease is still] curable.

【英译】

Line 290

[In] shaoyin [disease with] wind stroke, the yang pulse is faint and the yin pulse is floating, [indicating that the disease is] about to heal.

【原文】

(二九一)

少阴病欲解时,从子至寅上。

【今译】

少阴病解除的时间,大致从子时(晚上 11 时至凌晨 1 时)到寅时(凌晨 3 时至 5 时)。

【原文】

(二九二)

少阴病,吐,利,手足不逆冷,反发热者,不死。脉不至者,灸少阴七壮。

【今译】

少阴病中,患者呕吐,腹泻,手足不逆冷,反而发热,不会导致死亡。如果脉象不明,可用七壮艾条灸治少阴病。

【原文】

(二九三)

少阴病,八九日,一身手足尽热者,以热在膀胱,必便血也。

【今译】

少阴病患者,到了八九日,全身和手足都会发热,这是热在膀胱的缘故,必将导致小便下血。

Differentiation of pulse and syndrome/pattern [related to] shaoyin disease and treatment

【英译】

Line 291

The time to resolve shaoyin disease is about from zi (23:00 – 1:00) to yin (3:00 – 5:00).

【英译】

Line 292

[In] shaoyin disease, [although there are symptoms and signs of] vomiting, diarrhea and reversal cold of hands and feet, [there is still] fever, [so it will] not [lead to] death. [If] the pulse is not sensible, moxibustion [can be used to heat the acupoints located on] shaoyin [meridian] with seven cones of moxa.

【英译】

Line 293

[In] shaoyin disease, eight or nine days [after occurrence], [there are symptoms and signs of] fever over the whole body including hands and feet because [there is] heat in the bladder. [As a result,] hematuria will be caused.

【原文】

（二九四）

少阴病，但厥，无汗，而强发之，必动其血。未知从何道出，或从口鼻，或从目出者，是名下厥上竭，为难治。

【今译】

少阴病，唯有四肢厥冷和无汗等症状，如果强行发汗，必然导致出血，而出血部位则难以预测，或者从鼻孔出，或者从眼睛出，因此称为下厥上竭，为难治之症。

【原文】

（二九五）

少阴病，恶寒，身蜷而利，手足逆冷者，不治。

【今译】

少阴病，患者恶寒，踡卧，腹泻，手足逆冷，很难治疗。

【原文】

（二九六）

少阴病，吐，利，躁烦，四逆者，死。

【今译】

少阴病，患者呕吐，腹泻，烦躁，四肢逆冷的，为不治之症。

Differentiation of pulse and syndrome/pattern [related to] shaoyin disease and treatment

【英译】

Line 294

[In] shaoyin disease, [there are] only [symptoms and signs of] reversal cold of limbs and absence of sweating. If diaphoresis is forced [to use], [it will] inevitably cause hemorrhage, either from the nose or from the eyes, termed as lower coldness and upper exhaustion, very difficult to treat.

【英译】

Line 295

[In] shaoyin disease, [there are symptoms and signs of] aversion to cold, curling up when lying in bed, diarrhea and reversal cold of hands and feet, [indicating that the disease is] very difficult to treat.

【英译】

Line 296

[In] shaoyin disease, [there are symptoms and signs of] vomiting, diarrhea, vexation and coldness of the four limbs, [indicating that the disease is] not curable.

【原文】

(二九七)

少阴病,下利止而头眩,时时自冒者,死。

【今译】

少阴病,患者腹泻停止,但头部却眩晕,且时时自冒,为死症。

【原文】

(二九八)

少阴病,四逆,恶寒而身蜷,脉不至,不烦而躁者,死。

【今译】

少阴病,患者有四逆、恶寒、身蜷、脉不至、不烦而躁等症状的,为不治之症。

【原文】

(二九九)

少阴病,六七日,息高者,死。

【今译】

少阴病发作六七日后,患者呼吸困难,为不治之症。

Differentiation of pulse and syndrome/pattern
[related to] shaoyin disease and treatment

【英译】

Line 297

[In] shaoyin disease, diarrhea ceases, but [there is] dizziness and the vision is frequently dim, [indicating that it is] fatal.

【英译】

Line 298

[In] shaoyin disease, [there are symptoms and signs of] reversal [coldness in] the four [limbs], aversion to cold, curling up when lying in bed, insensible pulse, no vexation but restlessness, [indicating that the disease is] not curable.

【英译】

Line 299

Six or seven days [after occurrence of] shaoyin disease, [if the patient feels] very difficult to breathe, [it will cause] death.

【原文】

(三〇〇)

少阴病,脉微细沉,但欲卧,汗出不烦,自欲吐,至五六日,自利,复烦躁不得卧寐者,死。

【今译】

少阴病,患者脉微细沉,只想躺卧,汗出而不烦,想呕吐。五六日后,如果出现腹泻,再有烦躁,无法躺卧入睡的,为死症。

【原文】

(三〇一)

少阴病,初得之,反发热,脉沉者,麻黄细辛附子汤主之。

麻黄细辛附子汤方

麻黄二两(去节)、细辛二两、附子一枚(炮、去皮、破八片)。

右三味,以水一斗,先煮麻黄,减两升,去上沫,内诸药,煮取三升,去滓,温服一升,日三服。

【今译】

少阴病,刚开始发作时,反而发热,且脉象沉,宜用麻黄细辛附子汤主治。

Differentiation of pulse and syndrome/pattern [related to] shaoyin disease and treatment

【英译】

Line 300

[In] shaoyin disease, the pulse is faint, thin and sunken, [the patient] only wants to lie, [but there are symptoms and signs of] sweating, no vexation and desire to vomit. Five or six days later, [if there are still symptoms and signs of] diarrhea, relapse of vexation and difficulty to sleep, [it is] fatal.

【英译】

Line 301

[When] shaoyin disease has just occurred, [there is] fever and the pulse is sunken. Mahuang Xixin Fuzi Decoction (麻黄细辛附子汤, ephedra, asarum and aconite decoction) [can be used] to treat it.

Mahuang Xixin Fuzi Decoction (麻黄细辛附子汤, ephedra, asarum and aconite decoction) [is composed of] 2 *liang* of Mahuang (麻黄, ephedra, Herba Ephedrae) (remove the nodes), 2 *liang* of Xixin (细辛, asarum, Herba Asari) and 1 piece of Fuzi (附子, aconite, Radix Aconiti Lateralis Preparata) (fry heavily, remove the peel, and break into eight small pieces).

These three ingredients are decocted in 1 *dou* of water. Mahuang (麻黄, ephedra, Herba Ephedrae) (remove the nodes) is boiled first to reduce 2 *sheng* of water. The foam is removed and the other two ingredients are put into [it] to boil and get 3 *sheng*. The dregs are removed and [the decoction is] taken 1 *sheng* warm [each time] and three times a day.

【原文】

(三〇二)

少阴病,得之二三日,麻黄附子甘草汤微发汗,以二三日无证,故微发汗也。

麻黄附子甘草汤方

麻黄二两(去节)、甘草二两(炙)、附子一枚(炮,去皮,破八片)。

右三味,以水七升,先煮麻黄一两沸,去上沫,内诸药,煮取三升,去滓,温服一升,日三服。

【今译】

少阴病,发作两三天后,可用麻黄附子甘草汤微微发汗以解表。因为发病两三天时尚无吐、利等症状,所以通过微微发汗以解表。

【原文】

(三〇三)

少阴病,得之二三日以上,心中烦,不得卧,黄连阿胶汤主之。

黄连阿胶汤方

黄连四两、黄芩二两、芍药二两、鸡子黄二枚、阿胶三两(一云三挺)。

右五味,以水五升,先煮三物,取二升,去滓,内胶烊尽,小冷,内鸡子黄,搅令相得,温服七合,日三服。

【今译】

少阴病,发作两三天以上,患者心中烦躁不安,不能够安卧的,宜用黄连阿胶汤主治。

Differentiation of pulse and syndrome/pattern [related to] shaoyin disease and treatment

【英译】

Line 302

Two or three days [after occurrence of] shaoyin disease, Mahuang Fuzi Gancao Decoction (麻黄附子甘草汤, ephedra, aconite and licorice decoction) [can be used to induce] slight sweating. Because [the disease has occurred just for] two or three days, [there are] no symptoms and signs [like vomiting and diarrhea]. That is why sweating [should be induced] slightly.

Mahuang Fuzi Gancao Decoction (麻黄附子甘草汤, ephedra, aconite and licorice decoction) [is composed of] 2 *liang* of Mahuang (麻黄, ephedra, Herba Ephedrae) (remove the nodes), 2 *liang* of Gancao (甘草, licorice, Radix Glycyrrhizae Praeparata) (broil) and 1 piece of Fuzi (附子, aconite, Radix Aconiti Lateralis Preparata) (fry heavily, remove the peel, and break into eight small pieces).

These three ingredients are decocted in 7 *sheng* of water. Mahuang (麻黄, ephedra, Herba Ephedrae) (remove the nodes) is boiled first for once or twice. The foam is removed and the other two ingredients are put into [it] to boil and get 3 *sheng*. The dregs are removed and [the decoction is] taken 1 *sheng* warm [each time] and three times a day.

【英译】

Line 303

Over two or three days [after occurrence of] shaoyin disease, [the patient feels] vexing in the heart and unable to lie in bed. Huanglian Ejiao Decoction (黄连阿胶汤, coptis and ass-hide glue decoction) [can be used] to treat it.

Huanglian Ejiao Decoction (黄连阿胶汤, coptis and ass-hide glue decoction) [is composed of] 4 *liang* of Huanglian (黄连, coptis, Rhizoma Coptidis), 2 *liang* of Huangqin (黄芩, scutellaria, Radix Scutellariae), 2 pieces of Jizihuang (鸡子黄, egg yolk, Galli Vitellus) and 3 *liang* of Ejiao (阿胶, ass-hide glue, Colla Corii Asini).

These five ingredients are decocted in 5 *sheng* of water. Three ingredients are boiled first to get 2 *sheng*. The dregs are removed and Jizihuang (鸡子黄, egg yolk, Galli Vitellus) is put into [it] to dissolve completely. [When the decoction becomes] a little cooler, Jizihuang (鸡子黄, egg yolk, Galli Vitellus) is put into [it] and mixes [with other ingredients in the decoction]. [The decoction is] taken 7 *ge* warm [each time] and three times a day.

【原文】

(三〇四)

少阴病,得之一二日,口中和,其背恶寒者,当灸之,附子汤主之。

附子汤方

附子两枚(炮、去皮、破八片)、茯苓三两、人参二两、白术四两、芍药三两。

右五味,以水八升,煮取三升,去滓,温服一升,日三服。

【今译】

少阴病发作两三天后,患者口中无不适之感,但背部却怕冷,可用灸法解寒,宜用附子汤主治。

【原文】

(三〇五)

少阴病,身体痛,手足寒,骨节痛,脉沉者,附子汤主之。

【今译】

少阴病,身体疼痛,手足有冷感,关节疼痛,脉象沉,宜用附子汤主治。

Differentiation of pulse and syndrome/pattern [related to] shaoyin disease and treatment

【英译】

Line 304

One or two days [after occurrence of] shaoyin disease，[there is] no special taste in the mouth，but there is aversion to cold in the back，moxibustion [can be used to resolve] it. Fuzi Decoction (附子汤，aconite decoction) [can be used] to treat it.

Fuzi Decoction (附子汤，aconite decoction) [is composed of] 2 pieces of Fuzi (附子，aconite，Radix Aconiti Lateralis Preparata) (fry heavily，remove the peel and break into eight small pieces)，3 *liang* of Fuling (茯苓，poria，Poria)，2 *liang* of Renshen (人参，ginseng，Radix Ginseng)，4 *liang* of Baizhu (白术，rhizome of largehead atractylodes，Rhizoma Atractylodes Macrocephala) and 3 *liang* of Shaoyao (芍药，peony，Radix Paeoniae).

These five ingredients are decocted in 8 *sheng* of water to get 3 *sheng* [after] boiling. The dregs are removed and [the decoction is] taken warm 1 *sheng* [each time] and three times a day.

【英译】

Line 305

[In] shaoyin disease，[there are symptoms and signs of] generalized pain，cold hands and feet，arthralgia and sunken pulse. [It can be] treated by Fuzi Decoction (附子汤，aconite decoction).

【原文】

(三〇六)

少阴病,下利,便脓血者,桃花汤主之。

桃花汤方

赤石脂一斤(一半全用,一半筛末)、干姜一两、粳米一升。

右三味,以水七升,煮米令熟,去滓,温服七合,内赤石脂末方寸匕,日三服。若一服愈,余勿服。

【今译】

少阴病,患者腹泻而有脓血的,用桃花汤治疗。

【原文】

(三〇七)

少阴病,二三日至四五日,腹痛,小便不利,下利不止,便脓血者,桃花汤主之。

【今译】

少阴病发作两三天至四五天后,患者腹痛,小便不畅,腹泻不止,大便有脓血,用桃花汤主治。

Differentiation of pulse and syndrome/pattern [related to] shaoyin disease and treatment

【英译】

Line 306

[In] shaoyin disease, [there is] diarrhea with pus and blood. Taohua Decoction (桃花汤, peach blossom decoction) [can be used] to treat it.

Taohua Decoction (桃花汤, peach blossom decoction) [is composed of] 1 *jin* of Chishizhi (赤石脂, halloysite, Halloysitum Rubrum), 1 *liang* of Ganjiang (干姜, dried ginger, Rhizoma Zingiberis) and 1 *sheng* of Jingmi (粳米, polished round-grained rice, Semen Oryzae Sativae).

These three ingredients are decocted in 7 *sheng* of water. [When] rice is well boiled, the dregs are removed. [The decoction is] taken warm 7 *ge* [each time] and three times a day after 1 *fangcunbi* (about 1 gram) is mixed in it. If [the patient is] cured after taking one [dose], the rest [of the decoction is] forbidden to take.

【英译】

Line 307

[In] shaoyin disease, from two or three to four or five days [after occurrence], [there are symptoms and signs of] abdominal pain, dysuria, frequent diarrhea and stool with pus and blood. Taohua Decoction (桃花汤, peach blossom decoction) [can be used] to treat it.

【原文】

(三〇八)

少阴病,下利,便脓血者,可刺。

【今译】

少阴病,患者有腹泻、便脓血症状的,可用针刺法治疗。

【原文】

(三〇九)

少阴病,吐利,手足逆冷,烦躁欲死者,吴茱萸汤主之。

【今译】

少阴病,患者呕吐,腹泻,手足发凉,极度烦躁不安,以致有欲死之感,用吴茱萸汤主治。

【原文】

(三一〇)

少阴病,下利,咽痛,胸满,心烦,猪肤汤主之。

猪肤汤方

猪肤一斤。

Differentiation of pulse and syndrome/pattern [related to] shaoyin disease and treatment

【英译】

Line 308

[In] shaoyin disease，[there are symptoms and signs of] diarrhea and stool with pus and blood. [It] can [be treated by] acupuncture.

【英译】

Line 309

[In] shaoyin disease，[there are symptoms and signs of] vomiting，diarrhea，reversal cold of hands and feet，extreme vexation and severity about to die. Wuzhuyu Decoction（吴茱萸汤，evodia decoction）[can be used] to treat it.

【英译】

Line 310

[In] shaoyin disease，[there are symptoms and signs of] diarrhea，sore-throat，chest fullness and vexation. Zhufu Decoction（猪肤汤，pig skin decoction）[can be used] to treat it.

Zhufu Decoction（猪肤汤，pig skin decoction）[is composed of] 1 *jin* of Zhufu（猪肤，pig skin，Suis Corium）. This ingredient is decocted in 1 *dou* of water to get 5 *sheng* [after] boiling. [After] removal of the dregs，1 *sheng* of white honey and 5 *ge* of white

右一味,以水一斗,煮取五升,去滓,加白蜜一升,白粉五合,熬香,和令相得,温分六服。

【今译】

少阴病,患者腹泻,咽喉肿痛,胸部胀满,心中烦闷,用猪肤汤治疗。

【原文】

(三一一)

少阴病,二三日,咽痛者,可与甘草汤。不差者,与桔梗汤。

甘草汤方

甘草二两。

右一味,以水三升,煮取一升半,去滓,温服七合,日两服。

桔梗汤方

桔梗一两,甘草二两。

右二味,以水三升,煮取一升,去滓,温分再服。

【今译】

少阴病发作二三日后,患者有咽喉肿痛的,可用甘草汤治疗。如果没有治愈,可再用桔梗汤治疗。

powder are added to boil, making it aromatic and bending thoroughly. [The decoction is] divided into six [doses] and taken warm.

【英译】

Line 311

Two or three days [after occurrence of] shaoyin disease, [there is] sore-throat. [It] can be treated by Gancao Decoction (甘草汤, licorice decoction). [If it is] not cured, Jiegeng Decoction (桔梗汤, platy grandiforum decoction) [can be used] to treat [it].

Gancao Decoction (甘草汤, licorice decoction) [is composed of] 2 *liang* of Gancao (甘草, licorice, Radix Glycyrrhizae Praeparata). This ingredient is decocted in 3 *sheng* of water to get 1. 5 *sheng* [after] boiling. The dregs are removed and [the decoction is] taken 7 *ge* warm [each time] and twice a day.

Jiegeng Decoction (桔梗汤, platycodon grandiflorum decoction) [is composed of] 1 *liang* of Jiegeng (桔梗, platycodon grandiflorum, Radix Platycodi) and Gancao (甘草, licorice, Radix Glycyrrhizae Praeparata). These two ingredients are decocted in 3 *sheng* of water and get 1 *sheng* [after] boiling. The dregs are removed and [the decoction is] divided [into two doses] and taken warm.

【原文】

(三一二)

少阴病,咽中伤,生疮,不能语言。声不出者,苦酒汤主之。

苦酒汤方

半夏十四枚(洗,破如枣核)、鸡子一枚(去黄,内上苦酒,着鸡子壳中)。

右二味,内半夏,着苦酒中,以鸡子壳置刀环中,安火上,令三沸,去滓,少少含咽之。不差,更作三剂。

【今译】

少阴病,患者咽喉受伤,发生破溃,不能言语,说话发不出声音,可用苦酒汤治疗。

【原文】

(三一三)

少阴病,咽中痛,半夏散及汤主之。

半夏散及汤方

半夏(洗)、桂枝(去皮)、甘草(炙)。

右三味,等分,各别捣筛已,合治之,白饮和,服方寸匕,日三服。若不能服散者,以水一升,煎七沸,内散两方寸匕;更煮三沸,下火令小冷,少少咽之。半夏有毒,不当散服。

【今译】

少阴病,患者咽喉肿痛,可用半夏散及半夏汤治疗。

Differentiation of pulse and syndrome/pattern [related to] shaoyin disease and treatment

【英译】

Line 312

[In] shaoyin disease, [the patient suffers from] injury of the throat with sores, inability to speak and no voice in speaking. Kujiu Decoction (苦酒汤, bitter wine decoction) [can be used] to treat it.

Kujiu Decoction (苦酒汤, bitter wine decoction) [is composed of] 14 pieces of Banxia (半夏, pinellia, Rhizoma Pinelliae) (wash and break into pieces like kernel of jujube), 1 piece of Jizi (鸡子, chicken egg, Ovum Galli) (remove yolk, pour bitter wine into the egg shell).

Among these two ingredients, Banxia (半夏, pinellia, Rhizoma Pinelliae) is soaked in bitter wine and Jizi (鸡子, chicken egg, Ovum Galli) is put on the ring of a knife over fire and boiled for three times. The dregs are removed and [the decoction is] taken just a little, keeping [it in the mouth for a while and then] swallowing it. [If the disease is] not cured, [the patient can] take three more doses.

【英译】

Line 313

[In] shaoyin disease, [the patient suffers from] sore-throat. Banxia Powder and Decoction (半夏散及汤, pinellia powder and decoction) [can be used] to treat it.

Banxia Powder and Decoction (半夏散及汤, pinellia powder and decoction) [is composed of] Banxia (半夏, pinellia, Rhizoma Pinelliae) (wash), Guizhi (桂枝, cinnamon twig, Ramulus Cinnamomi) (remove the bark) and Gancao (甘草, licorice, Radix Glycyrrhizae Praeparata) (broil).

These three ingredients are of the same dose, pounded and sieved separately, and mixed with each other. [The decoction is] taken 1 *fangcunbi* (about 1 gram) [each time] and three times a day. If [the patient] cannot take the powder, [it should be] boiled in 1 *sheng* of water for seven times with 2 *fangcunbi* (about 2 grams) of powder [put in it]. [It is] boiled for three more times, removed from fire to cool for a while and swallowed a little [each time]. Banxia (半夏, pinellia, Rhizoma Pinelliae) is poisonous and should not be taken in powder.

【原文】

(三一四)

少阴病,下利,白通汤主之。

白通汤方

葱白四茎、干姜一两、附子一枚(生,去皮,破八片)。

右三味,以水三升,煮取一升,去滓,分温再服。

【今译】

少阴病,患者腹泻,可用白通汤治疗。

【原文】

(三一五)

少阴病,下利,脉微者,与白通汤。利不止,厥逆无脉,干呕,烦者,白通加猪胆汁汤主之。服汤,脉暴出者死,微续者生。

白通加猪胆汁汤方

葱白四茎、干姜一两、附子一枚(生,去皮,破八片)、人尿五合、猪胆汁一合。

右五味,以水三升,煮取一升,去滓,内胆汁、人尿,和令相得,分温再服。若无胆亦可用。

【今译】

少阴病,患者腹泻,脉象微的,可用白通汤治疗。若服药后腹泻不止,四肢逆冷,摸不到脉,干呕,烦躁不安的,可用白通加猪胆汁汤治疗。服药后,脉搏突然暴现的,预后不良;脉搏逐渐恢复的,预后良好。

Differentiation of pulse and syndrome/pattern [related to] shaoyin disease and treatment

【英译】

Line 314

[In] shaoyin disease, [the patient suffers from] diarrhea. Baitong Decoction (白通汤, scallion decoction for freeing yang) [can be used] to treat it.

Baitong Decoction (白通汤, scallion decoction for freeing yang) [is composed of] 4 stems of Congbai (葱白, white rhizome of Chinese scallion, Caulis Alli Fistulosi), 1 *liang* of Ganjiang (干姜, dried ginger, Rhizoma Zingiberis) and 1 piece of Fuzi (附子, aconite, Radix Aconiti Lateralis Preparata) (raw, remove the peel and break into eight small pieces).

These three ingredients are decocted in 3 *sheng* of water to get 1 *sheng* [after] boiling. The dregs are removed and [the decoction is] divided [into two doses] and taken warm.

【英译】

Line 315

[In] shaoyin disease, [there is] diarrhea with faint pulse, Baitong Decoction (白通汤, scallion decoction for freeing yang) [can be used] to treat [it]. [If] diarrhea is incessant, [and there is] reversal cold of limbs with dry retching, [it can be] treated by Baitong Decoction (白通汤, scallion decoction for freeing yang) added with Zhudanzhi Decoction (猪胆汁汤, pig's bile decoction). [If] the pulse suddenly begins to beat rapidly [after taking the decoction], [it is] fatal; [if the pulse] gradually starts to move mildly, [it is] curable.

Baitong Decoction (白通汤, scallion decoction for freeing yang) added with Zhudanzhi Decoction (猪胆汁汤, pig's bile decoction) [is composed of] 4 stems of Congbai (葱白, white rhizome of Chinese scallion, Bulbus Allii Fistulosi), 1 *liang* of Ganjiang (干姜, dried ginger, Rhizoma Zingiberis), 1 piece of Fuzi (附子, aconite, Radix Aconiti Lateralis Preparata) (raw, remove the peel and break into eight small pieces), 5 *ge* of Renniao (人尿, human urine, Huminis Urina) and 1 *ge* of Zhudanzhi (猪胆汁, pig's bile, Suis Bilis).

These five ingredients are decocted in 3 *sheng* of water to get 1 *sheng* [after] boiling. The dregs are removed, pig's bile and human urine are added to blend thoroughly. [The decoction is] divided [into two doses] and taken warm. If there is no [pig's] bile, [the formula] still can be used.

【原文】

(三一六)

少阴病,二三日不已,至四五日,腹痛,小便不利,四肢沉重疼痛,自下利者,此为有水气。其人或咳,或小便利,或下利,或呕者,真武汤主之。

真武汤方

茯苓三两、芍药三两、白术二两、生姜三两(切)、附子一枚(炮,去皮,破八片)。

右五味,以水八升,煮取三升,去滓,温服七合,日三服。若咳者,加五味子半升,细辛一两,干姜一两。若小便利者,去茯苓。若下利者,去芍药,加干姜二两。若呕者,去附子,加生姜,足前为半斤。

【今译】

少阴病,两三天后还未治好,到了四五天后,患者出现腹中疼痛,小便不畅,四肢沉重又疼痛,腹泻的,这是水气泛滥所致。患者出现或咳嗽,或小便通畅,或者腹泻严重,或呕吐等症状等,用真武汤主治。

Differentiation of pulse and syndrome / pattern [related to] shaoyin disease and treatment

【英译】

Line 316

[When] shaoyin disease is not cured in two or three days [after occurrence], at the fourth or fifth day, [there will appear] abdominal pain, inhibited urination, heaviness and pain of the four limbs and spontaneous diarrhea. This is caused by [flooding of] water qi. The patient [may suffer from] either cough, or normal urination, or severe diarrhea, or retching. [It can be] treated by Zhenwu Decoction (真武汤, true warrior decoction).

Zhenwu Decoction (真武汤, true warrior decoction) [is composed of] 3 *liang* of Fuling (茯苓, poria, Poria), 3 *liang* of Shaoyao (芍药, peony, Radix Paeoniae), 2 *liang* of Baizhu (白术, rhizome of largeheaded atractylode, Rhizoma Atractylodes Macrocephala), 3 *liang* of Shengjiang (生姜, fresh ginger, Rhizoma Zingiberis Recens) (cut) and 1 piece of Fuzi (附子, aconite, Radix Aconiti Lateralis Preparata) (fry heavily, remove the peel and break into eight small pieces).

These five ingredients are decocted in 8 *sheng* of water to get 3 *sheng* [after] boiling. The dregs are removed and [the decoction is] taken warm 7 ge [each time] and three times a day. If [there is] cough, 0.5 *sheng* of Wuweizi (五味子, schisandra, Fructus Schisandrae), 1 *liang* of Xixin (细辛, asarum, Herba Asari) and 1 *liang* of Ganjiang (干姜, dried ginger, Rhizoma Zingiberis) are added. If urination is uninhibited, Fuling (茯苓, poria, Poria) [should be] removed. If [there is] diarrhea, Shaoyao (芍药, peony, Radix Paeoniae) is removed and 2 *liang* of Ganjiang (干姜, dried ginger, Rhizoma Zingiberis) is added. If [there is] retching, Fuzi (附子, aconite, Radix Aconiti Lateralis Preparata) is removed and Shengjiang (生姜, fresh ginger, Rhizoma Zingiberis Recens) is added to 0.5 *jin*.

【原文】

(三一七)

少阴病,下利清谷,里寒外热,手足厥逆,脉微欲絶,身反不恶寒,其人面色赤,或腹痛,或干呕,或咽痛,或利止脉不出者,通脉四逆汤主之。

通脉四逆汤方

甘草二两(炙)、附子大者一枚(生用,去皮,破八片)、干姜三两,强人可四两。

右三味,以水三升,煮取一升二合,去滓,分温再服,其脉即出者愈。面色赤者,加葱九茎。腹中痛者,去葱,加芍药二两。呕者,加生姜二两。咽痛者,去芍药,加桔梗一两。利止脉不出者,去桔梗,加人参二两。病皆与方相应者,乃服之。

【今译】

少阴病,腹泻完谷不化,体内感到寒冷,体外感到闷热,手足冰冷,脉象微弱的是没有搏动,但身上反而不怕冷,病人面部发红,或者腹中疼痛,或者干呕,或者咽喉疼痛,或者腹泻不止,甚至摸不到脉搏,用通脉四逆汤主治。

Differentiation of pulse and syndrome/pattern [related to] shaoyin disease and treatment

【英译】

Line 317

Shaoyin disease [is characterized by] diarrhea with undigested food, internal cold and external heat, reversal cold of hands and feet, faint pulse almost unmovable, absence of aversion to cold, reddish facial expression, or abdominal pain, or dry retching, or sore-throat, or unmovable pulse [when] diarrhea has ceased. Tongmai Sini Decoction (通脉四逆汤, decoction for freeing vessels and resolving four kinds of adverseness) [can be used] to treat it.

Tongmai Sini Decoction (通脉四逆汤, decoction for freeing vessels and resolving four kinds of adverseness) [is composed of] 2 *liang* of Gancao (甘草, fried licorice, Radix Glycyrrhizae Praeparata) (broil), 1 piece of Fuzi (附子, aconite, Radix Aconiti Lateralis Preparata) (raw, remove the peel and break into eight small pieces) and 3 *liang* of Ganjiang (干姜, dried ginger, Rhizoma Zingiberis) or 4 *liang* [if] the patient is strong.

These three ingredients are decocted in 3 *sheng* of water to get 1 *sheng* and 2 *ge* [after] boiling. The dregs are removed and [the decoction is] divided [into two doses] and taken warm. [When] the pulse moves, [the disease will] heal. For reddish facial expression, add 9 stems of Congbai (葱白, white rhizome of Chinese scallion, Bulbus Allii Fistulosi); for abdominal pain, remove Congbai (葱白, white rhizome of Chinese scallion, Bulbus Allii Fistulosi), add 2 *liang* of Shaoyao (芍药, peony, Radix Paeoniae); for diarrhea, add 2 *liang* of Shengjiang (生姜, fresh ginger, Rhizoma Zingiberis Recens); for sore-throat, remove Shaoyao (芍药, peony, Radix Paeoniae), add 1 *liang* of Jiegeng (桔梗, platycodon grandiflorum, Radix Platycodonis); for unmovable pulse when diarrhea has ceased, remove Jiegeng (桔梗, platycodon grandiflorum, Radix Platycodonis), add 2 *liang* of Renshen (人参, ginseng, Radix Ginseng). [The decoction] can be taken [only when the manifestations of] the disease correspond to the formula.

【原文】

(三一八)

少阴病,四逆,其人或欬,或悸,或小便不利,或腹中痛,或泄利下重者,四逆散主之。

四逆散方

甘草(炙)、枳实(破,水渍,炙干)、柴胡、芍药。

右四味,各十分,捣筛,白饮和服方寸匕,日三服。咳者,加五味子、干姜各五分,并主下利。悸者,加桂枝五分。小便不利者,加茯苓五分。腹中痛者,加附子一枚,炮令坼。泄利下重者,先以水五升,煮薤白三升,煮取三升,去滓,以散三方寸匕,内汤中,煮取一升半,分温再服。

【今译】

少阴病,四肢逆冷,病人或咳嗽,或心悸,或小便不畅,或腹中疼痛,或腹泻后重,宜用四逆散主治。

Differentiation of pulse and syndrome/pattern [related to] shaoyin disease and treatment

【英译】

Line 318

[In] shaoyin disease，[there is] reversal [cold of] the four [limbs]，the patient [suffers from] either cough，or palpitation，or inhibited urination，or abdominal pain，or diarrhea with heavy [feeling of] the rectum. Sini Powder（四逆散，powder for resolving four kinds of adverseness）[can be used] to treat it.

Sini Powder（四逆散，powder for resolving four kinds of adverseness）[is composed of] Gancao（甘草，licorice，Radix Glycyrrhizae Praeparata）（broil），Zhishi（枳实，unripe bitter orange，Fructus Aurantii Immaturus）（break，soak and broil dry），Chaihu（柴胡，bupleurum，Radix Bupleuri）and Shaoyao（芍药，peony，Radix Paeoniae）.

These four ingredients，10 *fen* each，are pounded，sieved and mixed in boiled water or porridge. [It is] taken one *fangcunbi* （about 1 gram）[each time and] three times a day. For cough，add 5 *fen* of Wuweizi（五味子，schisandra，Fructus Schisandrae Chinensis）and 1 *liang* of Ganjiang（干姜，dried ginger，Rhizoma Zingiberis），also dealing with diarrhea. For palpitation，add 5 *fen* of Guizhi（桂枝，cinnamon twig，Ramulus Cinnamomi）. For inhibited urination，add 5 *fen* of Fuling（茯苓，poria，Poria）. For abdominal pain，add 1 piece of Fuzi（附子，aconite，Radix Aconiti Lateralis Preparata）[which is] fried and cracked. For diarrhea with heavy [feeling of] the rectum，boil 3 *sheng* of Xiebai（薤白，longstamen onion bulb，Bulbus Allii Macrostemonis）in 5 *sheng* of water to get 3 *sheng*，remove the dregs，put 3 *fangcunbi*（3 grams）of the powder in the decoction to get 1. 5 *sheng* [after] boiling，divide [into two doses] and take warm.

【原文】

(三一九)

少阴病,下利六七日,咳而呕渴,心烦不得眠者,猪苓汤主之。

猪苓汤方

猪苓(去皮)、茯苓、泽泻、阿胶、滑石(碎)各一两。

右五味,以水四升,先煮四味,取两升,去滓,内阿胶烊消,温服七合,日三服。

【今译】

少阴病,腹泻六七天后,患者咳嗽,呕吐,口渴,心中烦躁,不能安眠,用猪苓汤主治。

【原文】

(三二〇)

少阴病,得之二三日,口燥,咽干者,急下之,宜大承气汤。

【今译】

少阴病,发作两三天后,患者口燥,咽喉干。应采用急下法治疗,宜用大承气汤主治。

Differentiation of pulse and syndrome/pattern [related to] shaoyin disease and treatment

【英译】

Line 319

[In] shaoyin disease, six or seven days [after] diarrhea, [there are symptoms and signs of] cough, vomiting, thirst, vexation and inability to sleep. Zhuling Decoction (猪苓汤, polyporus powder) [can be used] to treat it.

Zhuling Decoction (猪苓汤, polyporus decoction) [is composed of] 1 *liang* of Zhuling (猪苓, polyporus, Polyporus Umbellatus) (remove the peel), 1 *liang* of Fuling (茯苓, poria, Poria). 1 *liang* of Zexie (泽泻, alisma, Rhizoma Alismatis), 1 *liang* of Ejiao (阿胶, ass-hide glue, Colla Corri Asini) and 1 *liang* of Huashi (滑石, talcum, Talcum) (crush).

These five ingredients are decocted in 4 *sheng* of water. Four ingredients are boiled first to get 2 *sheng*. [When] the dregs are removed, Ejiao (阿胶, ass-hide glue, Colla Corri Asini) is put into it to melt. [The decoction is] taken warm 7 *ge* [each time] and three times a day.

【英译】

Line 320

Two or three days [after occurrence of] shaoyin disease, [there is] dryness of the mouth and throat. Drastic purgation [should be used]. The appropriate [formula] is Da Chengqi Decoction (大承气汤, major decoction for harmonizing qi).

【原文】

(三二一)

少阴病,自利清水,色纯青,心下必痛,口干燥者,可下之,宜大承气汤。

【今译】

少阴病,腹泻稀水,颜色纯青,脘腹疼痛,口中干燥,可用攻下法,宜以大承气汤主治。

【原文】

(三二二)

少阴病,六七日,腹胀,不大便者,急下之,宜大承气汤。

【今译】

少阴病发作六七日后,患者腹部胀满,大便不通,可用急下之法,宜用大承气汤主治。

Differentiation of pulse and syndrome / pattern [related to] shaoyin disease and treatment

【英译】

Line 321

Shaoyin disease, [characterized by] diarrhea with clear water pure and green in color, pain below the heart and dryness of the mouth, can [be treated by] purgation. The appropriate [formula is] Da Chengqi Decoction (大承气汤, major decoction for harmonizing qi).

【英译】

Line 322

[In] shaoyin disease, six or seven days [after occurrence], [there is] abdominal distension without defecation. Drastic purgation [can be used to treat] it. The appropriate [formula is] Da Chengqi Decoction (大承气汤, major decoction for harmonizing qi).

【原文】

(三二三)

少阴病,脉沉者,急温之,宜四逆汤。

四逆汤方

甘草二两(炙)、干姜一两、半附子一枚(生用,去皮,破八片)。

右三味,以水三升,煮取一升二合,去滓,分温再服。强人可大附子一枚,干姜三两。

【今译】

少阴病中脉沉的,应急用温法治疗,宜用四逆汤主治。

【原文】

(三二四)

少阴病,饮食入口则吐,心中温温欲吐,复不能吐,初得之,手足寒,脉弦迟者,此胸中实,不可下也,当吐之。若膈上有寒饮,干呕者,不可吐也,当温之,宜四逆汤。

【今译】

少阴病,患者饮食入口即吐,心中蕴结欲吐,但却吐不出,初得病时,手足寒冷,脉象弦迟,这是胸中邪实所致,不能攻下,应当用涌吐法治疗。如果寒饮停聚膈上,而导致干呕的,不能用涌吐法治疗,应用温法治疗,宜用四逆汤主治。

Differentiation of pulse and syndrome/pattern [related to] shaoyin disease and treatment

【英译】

Line 323

Shaoyin disease with sunken pulse should [be treated] immediately by warming [therapy]. The appropriate [formula is] Sini Decoction (四逆汤, decoction for resolving four kinds of adverseness).

Sini Decoction (四逆汤, decoction for resolving four kinds of adverseness [is composed of] 2 *liang* of Gancao (甘草, licorice, Radix Glycyrrhizae Praeparata) (broil), 1.5 *liang* of Ganjiang (干姜, dried ginger, Rhizoma Zingiberis) and 1 piece of Fuzi (附子, aconite, Radix Aconiti Lateralis Preprarata) (raw, remove the bark and break into 8 small pieces).

These three ingredients are decocted in 3 *sheng* of water to get 1 *sheng* and 2 *ge* [after] boiling. The dregs are removed and [the decoction is] divided [into two doses] and taken warm. [If] the patient is strong, 1 piece of Fuzi (附子, aconite, Radix Aconiti) and 3 *liang* of Ganjiang (干姜, dried ginger, Rhizoma Zingiberis) are added.

【英译】

Line 324

[In] shaoyin disease, [the patient] vomits [when] taking food and desires to vomit when the heart is seething, but is unable to vomit. At the beginning, [there are symptoms and signs of] cold hands and feet, taut and slow pulse due to [pathogenic] excess in the chest [which] must not be purged with vomiting [therapy]. If there is [retention of] cold fluid in the diaphragm with dry retching, [it should be treated by] warming [thereapy]. The appropriate [formula] is Sini Decoction (四逆汤, decoction for resolving four kinds of adverseness).

【原文】

(三二五)

少阴病,下利,脉微涩,呕而汗出,必数更衣,反少者,当温其上,灸之。

【今译】

少阴病,腹泻,脉微涩,呕吐又出汗,必然导致大便频频,但量反而少,应温热其上,可用灸法治疗。

Differentiation of pulse and syndrome / pattern [related to] shaoyin disease and treatment

【英译】

Line 325

[In] shaoyin disease, diarrhea, faint and rough pulse, vomiting and sweating will inevitably lead to frequent but scanty defecation. [To treat it,] the upper should be warmed with moxibustion.

辨厥阴病脉证并治

【原文】

(三二六)

厥阴之为病，消渴，气上撞心，心中疼热，饥而不欲食，食则吐蛔。下之利不止。

【今译】

厥阴病的主要症候，是口渴，气逆上冲心胸，心中灼热疼痛，腹中虽饿但却不想进食，如果进食就会呕吐或吐出蛔虫。如果误用了攻下法，就会使腹泻不止。

【原文】

(三二七)

厥阴中风，脉微浮为欲愈，不浮为未愈。

【今译】

厥阴中风病，脉象微浮，为疾病将愈的征兆。如果脉象不浮，即病还未愈。

Differentiation of pulse and syndrome/pattern [related to] jueyin disease and treatment

Differentiation of pulse and syndrome/pattern [related to] jueyin disease and treatment

【英译】

Line 326

Jueyin disease [is mainly characterized by] wasting-thirst, counterflow of qi against the heart, pain and heat in the chest, hunger without desire to eat, vomiting or vomiting of worms after taking food and diarrhea [if be treated by] purgation.

【英译】

Line 327

[In] jueyin [disease] with wind stroke, slightly floating pulse indicates [that the disease is] about to heal. [If the pulse is] not floating, [it] indicates [that the disease is] not cured.

【原文】

(三二八)

厥阴病,欲解时,从丑至卯上。

【今译】

厥阴病将解除的时间,一般从丑时(凌晨 1—3 点)到卯时(早上 5—7 点)。

【原文】

(三二九)

厥阴病,渴欲饮水者,少少与之愈。

【今译】

厥阴病,患者口渴想饮水,只有少量饮水才会使疾病逐步痊愈。

【原文】

(三三〇)

诸四逆厥者,不可下之,虚家亦然。

【今译】

各种四逆厥证,不可以用泻下法治疗,虚证也是如此。

Differentiation of pulse and syndrome/pattern [related to] jueyin disease and treatment

【英译】

Line 328

[The time that] jueyin disease is about to heal is usually from [the time of] chou (1:00 - 3:00) to [the time of] mao (5:00 - 7:00).

【英译】

Line 329

[In] jueyin disease, [the patient] wants to drink water. [But only when the patient drinks] a little water [each time can the disease eventually] heal.

【英译】

Line 330

[In all syndromes/patterns related to] reversal cold of limbs, no purgation can be used [to treat it], and so is deficiency [syndrome/pattern].

【原文】

(三三一)

伤寒,先厥,后发热而利者,必自止;见厥复利。

【今译】

伤寒病,先厥冷,后发热而腹泻,必然会自行停止。只要有厥冷,腹泻就会再现。

【原文】

(三三二)

伤寒,初发热六日,厥反九日而利。凡厥利者,当不能食;今反能食者,恐为除中。食以索饼,不发热者,知胃气尚在,必愈。恐暴热来出而复去也。后三日脉之,其热续在者,期之旦日夜半愈。所以然者,本发热六日,厥反九日,复发热三日,并前六日,亦为九日,与厥相应,故期之旦日夜半愈。后三日脉之而脉数,其热不罢者,此为热气有余,必发痈脓也。

【今译】

伤寒初起发热六天,接着四肢逆冷、大便泄泻持续达九天。四肢逆冷、大便泄泻的患者,按常理应该不能饮食,但现在的患者反而能饮食,可能是胃气将除的反应。这时可以给患者吃面饼类食物,吃后如果不发热,说明胃气尚存,其病必然痊愈。最担心的是患者吃饭后突然发热,体温又突然下降。后三天检查,如果微热仍在,明日半夜可将痊愈。为什么呢?因为本来发热六天,厥冷反而有九天,今又发热三天,加上以前六天,也是九天,和厥冷的天数相等,所以可以预测明天半夜痊愈。如果又过三天,复诊时脉搏急数,发热不退,这是热气太过,必然发生痈疮脓疡。

Differentiation of pulse and syndrome/pattern [related to] jueyin disease and treatment

【英译】

Line 331

[In] cold damage [disease], reversal [cold] first [occurs], the following is fever with diarrhea [which will] spontaneously cease. [When] there is cold, [there will be] diarrhea again.

【英译】

Line 332

[In] cold damage [disease], [there is] heat [for] six days at the onset [of the disease], and [there are] reversal [cold of limbs] and diarrhea for nine days. [Usually patients with] reversal [cold of limbs] and diarrhea are unable to take food. But now [the patient] can take food, perhaps because [pathogenic factors in] stomach qi [will be] eliminated. [If the patient is asked] to eat cakes, and [if there is] no heat, [it] indicates that stomach qi is still present and [the disease will] heal. Great cares must be taken to avoid heat now suddenly occurring and then suddenly disappearing. In the next three days, examination may find that heat is still present, expecting recovery at the midnight the next day. The reason is that originally there is heat for six days and there is reversal [cold of limbs] for nine days. Now there is heat again for another three days, together with the previous six days, there is nine days, corresponding to [the nine days of] reversal [cold of limbs]. That is why recovery is expected at the midnight the next day. In the next three days, examination finds that the pulse is rapid and heat is still present, indicating that heat is excessive and inevitably causes abscess and ulceration.

【原文】

(三三三)

伤寒脉迟，六七日，而反与黄芩汤彻其热，脉迟为寒，今与黄芩汤复除其热，腹中应冷，当不能食，今反能食，此名除中，必死。

【今译】

伤寒病，患者脉迟，六七日后，反而用黄芩汤除其热。脉迟本属寒症，现在用黄芩汤再除其热，腹中应当寒冷，因此应当不能饮食，现在反而能饮食的，这种症候称为除中，必然导致死亡。

【原文】

(三三四)

伤寒，先厥后发热，下利必自止。而反汗出，咽中痛者，其喉为痹。发热无汗，而利必自止；若不止，必便脓血。便脓血者，其喉不痹。

【今译】

伤寒病，先见四肢厥冷，以后转为发热，腹泻必然自行停止。如果发热反见出汗、咽喉肿痛的，将产生喉痹。如果发热无汗，腹泻必然自行停止。如果腹泻不止的，必然会下利脓血。如果出现下利脓血，喉痹则不会发生。

Differentiation of pulse and syndrome/pattern [related to] jueyin disease and treatment

【英译】

Line 333

[In] cold damage [disease], the pulse is slow, six or seven days after [occurrence], Huangqin Decoction (黄芩汤, scutellaria decoction) is used to eliminate heat. Slow pulse originally indicates cold. Now Huangqin Decoction (黄芩汤, scutellaria decoction) is used to eliminate heat, there should be coldness in the abdomen and [the patient] should be unable to eat. But now [the patient is] able to eat. Such a syndrome/pattern is called elimination of the middle and is also fatal.

【英译】

Line 334

[In] cold damage [disease], there is first reversal [cold of limbs] and then fever. [As a result,] diarrhea will spontaneously cease. [If there is] no sweating in the presence of fever, diarrhea will spontaneously cease. If it does not cease, there will be stool with pus and blood. [If there is] stool with pus and blood, there will be impediment in the throat.

【原文】

（三三五）

伤寒，一二日至四五日，厥者必发热，前热者后必厥，厥深者热亦深，厥微者热亦微。厥应下之，而反发汗者，必口伤烂赤。

【今译】

伤寒病，发作一两日至四五日后，如四肢厥冷的，必然发热。如先发热而后四肢厥冷，厥冷严重的，热邪亦严重，厥冷轻微的，热邪也轻微。这种厥逆应用泻下法治疗，如果误用了汗法，势必引发口舌生疮、红肿糜烂。

【原文】

（三三六）

伤寒病，厥五日，热亦五日。设六日当复厥，不厥者自愈。厥终不过五日，以热五日，故知自愈。

【今译】

伤寒病，四肢厥冷五天，发热也是五天。到了第六天，四肢厥冷应当再次出现，若不出现则会自行痊愈。这是因为四肢厥冷持续只有五天，而发热也是五天，所以就会知道其自行痊愈。

Differentiation of pulse and syndrome/pattern [related to] jueyin disease and treatment

【英译】

Line 335

[In] cold damage [disease], one or two days to four or five days [after occurrence], [when there is] reveral [cold of limbs] there must be heat. [When there is] heat first, there must be reversal [cold of limbs] later. [When there is] severe reversal [cold of limbs], there must be severe heat. [When there is] slight reversal [cold of limbs], there must be slight heat. Coldness [of limbs] should [be treated by] purgation. If diaphoresis is used, it will cause oral sore and ulceration.

【英译】

Line 336

[In] cold damage [disease], [there is] reversal [cold of limbs] for five days, and so is heat. On the sixth day, there should be reversal [cold of limbs] again. [If there is] no reversal [cold of limbs], [the disease] will spontaneously heal. [The duration of] reversal [cold of limbs] will not surpass five days, and so will that of heat. That is why it is known [that the disease will] spontaneously heal.

【原文】

(三三七)

凡厥者,阴阳气不相顺接,便为厥。厥者,手足逆冷者是也。

【今译】

所有厥症,因阴气和阳气相互不能顺利交接而发生厥症。厥的主要表现为手足逆冷。

【原文】

(三三八)

伤寒,脉微而厥,至七八日肤冷,其人躁无暂安时者,此为脏厥,非蛔厥也。蛔厥者,其人当吐蛔,今病者静而复时烦者,此为脏寒,蛔上入其膈,故烦,须臾复止,得食而呕,又烦者,蛔闻食臭出,其人常自吐蛔。蛔厥者,乌梅丸主之。又主久利。

乌梅丸方

乌梅二百枚、细辛六两、干姜十两、黄连一斤、当归四两、附子六两(炮,去皮)、蜀椒四两(出汗)、桂枝六两(去皮)、人参六两、黄柏六两。

右十味,异捣筛,合治之,以苦酒渍乌梅一宿,去核,蒸之五升米下,饭熟捣成泥,和药令相得,内臼中,与蜜杵两千下,丸如梧桐子大。先食饮服十丸,日三服,稍加至二十丸,禁生冷、滑物、臭食等。

Differentiation of pulse and syndrome / pattern [related to] jueyin disease and treatment

【英译】

Line 337

In all [syndromes/patterns of] reversal [cold of limbs], yin and yang fail to connect with each other, causing reversal [cold of limbs]. Reversal [cold of limbs] refers to aversion to cold in the hands and feet.

【英译】

Line 338

[In] cold damage [disease], the pulse is faint and [there is] reversal [cold of limbs]. Seven or eight days [after occurrence], [there is] cold in the skin and the patient feels vexing and there is no temporary quiet. This is visceral reversal [cold], not worm reversal [cold]. [In case of] worm reversal [cold], the patient should vomit worms. But now the patient is quiet and [there is] periodic vexation. This is visceral coldness, [in which] worms enter the diaphragm. That is why [there is] vexation [which will] cease after a while. [After] taking food, [there will be] vomiting and vexation [because] worms have smelled malodor of food. [That is why] the patient often vomits worms. Worm reversal [cold can be] treated by Wumei Pill (乌梅丸, mume pill) [which can] also treat enduring diarrhea.

Wumei Pill (乌梅丸, mume pill) [is composed of] 200 pieces of Wumei (乌梅, mume, Fructus Mume), 6 *liang* of Xixin (细辛, asarum, Herba Asari), 10 *liang* of Ganjiang (干姜, dried ginger, Rhizoma Zingiberis), 1 *jin* of Huanglian (黄连, coptis, Rhizoma Coptidis), 4 *liang* of Danggui (当归, Chinese angelica, Radix Angelicae Sinensis), 6 *liang* of Fuzi (附子, aconite, Radix Aconiti

【今译】

伤寒病,脉象微而四肢厥冷,七八天后肌肤冰冷,患者烦躁,无片刻安静,这是脏厥证,并非蛔厥证。蛔厥证的患者呕吐应当有蛔虫。如今患者安静但心烦腹痛又时而发作,这是脏中有寒,蛔虫向上钻入膈内所致,所以烦躁,但过一会儿就会缓解。进餐后又呕吐,又烦闷的,是蛔虫闻到食物上扰所致。此外,病人常呕吐蛔虫。蛔厥证,可用乌梅丸治疗,还可治疗久泻。

【原文】

(三三九)

伤寒热少微厥,指头寒,嘿嘿不欲食,烦躁。数日,小便利,色白者,此热除也。欲得食,其病为愈;若厥而呕,胸胁烦满者,其后必便血。

【今译】

伤寒病,邪热较轻,四肢轻微厥冷,患者指头发凉,神情默默,不想进食,烦躁不安。几天之后,小便通畅,颜色清白,表明里热已除。此时患者如果想进食,说明病将痊愈。如果依然四肢厥冷而呕吐,胸胁满闷而烦躁,此后必将出现便血的病变。

Differentiation of pulse and syndrome / pattern [related to] jueyin disease and treatment

Lateralis Preparata) (fry heavily and remove the bark), 4 *liang* of Shujiao (蜀椒, zanthoxylum, Pericarpium Zanthoxyli), 6 *liang* of Guizhi (桂枝, cinnamon twig, Ramulus Cinnamomi) (remove the bark), 6 *liang* of Renshen (人参, ginseng, Radix Ginseng) and 6 *liang* of Huangbo (黄柏, phellodendron, Cortex Phellodendri).

These ten ingredients are pounded and sieved to combine with each other for treatment. The mume is soaked in bitter wine for one night. [When] the kernels are removed, [it is] steamed with 5 *sheng* of rice. [When] the rice is well cooked, [it is] pounded into paste and blended with medicinals. Put it into a mortar and pound it with honey for two thousand times, making the pills the size of firmiana seeds. Take ten pills before eating, three times a day, and gradually increasing to twenty pills [each time]. [It is] forbidden [to take] raw and cold [food], slimy and malodorous food [when taking the pills].

【英译】

Line 339

[In] cold damage [disease], heat is scanty and reversal [cold] is slight. [There are symptoms and signs of] cold fingers, taciturnity, no desire to eat and vexation. [After] several days, urine is uninhibited and clear, indicating elimination of heat. [If the patient] wants to eat, the disease is about to heal. If [there are symptoms and signs of] reversal [cold], retching, vexation and fullness in the chest and rib-side, there will be defecation with blood.

【原文】

(三四〇)

病者手足厥冷,言我不结胸,小腹满,按之痛者,此冷结在膀胱关元也。

【今译】

病人手足厥冷,自言胸部无痞痛,但小腹胀满,按之疼痛,这是由于寒气结在下焦所致。

【原文】

(三四一)

伤寒发热四日,厥反三日,复热四日,厥少热多者,其病当愈。四日至七日热不除者,必便脓血。

【今译】

伤寒病,发热四天,四肢厥冷三天,又发热四天,厥冷少而发热多,病应痊愈。如果到了第四天至第七天,发热仍不退,必然导致下利脓血。

Differentiation of pulse and syndrome/pattern [related to] jueyin disease and treatment

【英译】

Line 340

The patient's hands and feet are of reversal cold, saying [that there is] no lump and pain in the chest, [but there is] abdominal fullness [that feels] painful [when] pressed. This is caused by cold bind in the bladder and at Guanyuan (CV 4).

【英译】

Line 341

[In] cold damage [disease], there is heat for four days but reversal [cold of limbs] for three days. There is heat again for four more days. [The result is] more heat and less reversal [cold], [indicating that] the disease is about to heal. [From] the fourth day to the seventh day, [if] heat is not eliminated, there must be stool with pus and blood.

【原文】

(三四二)

伤寒厥四日,热反三日,复厥五日,其病为进。寒多热少,阳气退,故为进也。

【今译】

伤寒厥冷四日,发热仅三日,接着又厥冷五日,说明病势在进。寒多热少,表示阳气衰退,所以病势在进。

【原文】

(三四三)

伤寒六七日,脉微,手足厥冷,烦躁,灸厥阴,厥不还者,死。

【今译】

伤寒病发作了六七天,患者脉微,手足厥冷,烦躁不安,应灸厥阴经穴。如果灸后四肢厥冷仍不解,属死症。

【原文】

(三四四)

伤寒发热,下利,厥逆,躁不得卧者,死。

【今译】

伤寒病,患者发热,腹泻,手足厥冷。由于烦躁而不能安卧的,是死候。

Differentiation of pulse and syndrome/pattern [related to] jueyin disease and treatment

【英译】

Line 342

[In] cold damage [disease], [there is] reversal [cold of limbs] for four days, but [there is] heat just for three days. [Then there is] reversal [cold of limbs] again for five days, [indicating] progress of the disease. More coldness and less heat [indicate] debatement of yang qi. That is why [the disease] is progressing.

【英译】

Line 343

Six or seven days [after occurrence of] cold damage [disease], [there are symptoms and signs of] faint pulse, reversal cold of hands and feet and vexation. [Apply] moxibustion to jueyin [meridian]. [If] reversal [cold of limbs] is not resolved, [the disease is] fatal.

【英译】

Line 344

[In] cold damage [disease], [there are symptoms and signs of] fever, diarrhea and reversal cold of hands and feet. [If the patient] cannot sleep [because of] vexation, [it is] fatal.

【原文】

（三四五）

伤寒发热，下利至甚，厥不止者，死。

【今译】

伤寒病，发热，腹泻严重，四肢厥冷不止，属死候。

【原文】

（三四六）

伤寒六七日不利，便发热而利，其人汗出不止者，死。有阴无阳故也。

【今译】

伤寒病发作了六七日，原本没有腹泻，忽然发热腹泻，如果汗出不止的，属于死候，因为只有阴而没有阳。

【原文】

（三四七）

伤寒五六日，不结胸，腹濡，脉虚复厥者，不可下，此亡血，下之死。

【今译】

伤寒病发作五六天，无结胸症，腹部柔软，脉象虚软，四肢厥冷，不可用攻下法治疗，若误用攻下法，必然亡血，导致死亡。

Differentiation of pulse and syndrome/pattern [related to] jueyin disease and treatment

【英译】

Line 345

[In] cold damage [disease], [there are symptoms and signs of] fever, severe diarrhea and reversal [cold of limbs that] cannot cease, [it is] fatal.

【英译】

Line 346

[In] cold damage [disease], six or seven days [after occurrence], [originally there is] no diarrhea. But later on [there is] fever and diarrhea. [If there is] incessant sweating, [it is] fatal [because] there is only yin, but no yang.

【英译】

Line 347

[In] cold damage [disease], five or six days [after occurrence], [there is] no chest bind, the abdomen is soft, the pulse is weak and [the four limbs are of] reversal [cold] again. Purgation cannot [be used to treat it]. [If] used, [it will] cause blood collapse and death.

【原文】

(三四八)

发热而厥,七日下利者,为难治。

【今译】

发热而四肢厥冷,第七天又发生腹泻,为难治之症。

【原文】

(三四九)

伤寒脉促,手足厥逆,可灸之。

【今译】

伤寒病,脉象促,四肢厥冷,可用灸法治疗。

【原文】

(三五〇)

伤寒脉滑而厥者,里有热,白虎汤主之。

【今译】

伤寒病,脉象滑利,四肢厥冷,为里热所致,宜用白虎汤治疗。

Differentiation of pulse and syndrome/pattern [related to] jueyin disease and treatment

【英译】

Line 348

[In] cold damage [disease], [there is] fever and reversal [cold of limbs]. On the seventh day, [there is] diarrhea. [It is] very difficult to treat.

【英译】

Line 349

[In] cold damage [disease], the pulse is skipping, the hands and feet are of reversal cold. Moxibustion [can be used] to treat it.

【英译】

Line 350

[In] cold damage [disease], [there is] slippery pulse and reversal [cold of limbs], [indicating] heat in the internal. Baihu Decoction (白虎汤, white tiger decoction) [can be used] to treat it.

【原文】

(三五一)

手足厥寒,脉细欲绝者,当归四逆汤主之。

当时四逆汤方

当归三两、桂枝三两(去皮)、芍药三两、细辛三两、甘草二两(炙)、通草二两、大枣二十五枚(擘)(一法十二枚)。

右七味,以水八升,煮取三升,去滓,温服一升,日三服。

【今译】

伤寒病,手足厥冷,脉象细微,好似即将断绝一样,宜用当归四逆汤主治。

【原文】

(三五二)

若其人内有久寒者,宜当归四逆加吴茱萸生姜汤。

当归四逆加吴茱萸生姜汤方

当归二两、芍药三两、甘草二两(炙)、通草二两、桂枝三两(去皮)、细辛三两、生姜半斤(切)、吴茱萸二升、大枣二十五枚(擘)。

右九味,以水六升,清酒六升和,煮取五升,去滓,温分五服。一方水酒各四升。

【今译】

如果患者素有内寒,宜用当归四逆加吴茱萸生姜汤治疗。

Differentiation of pulse and syndrome/pattern [related to] jueyin disease and treatment

【英译】

Line 351

[In cold damage disease, there is] reversal cold of hands and feet and thin pulse [that seems] on the verge of expiry. Danggui Sini Decoction (当归四逆汤, Chinese angelica decoction for resolving four kinds of adverseness) [can be used] to treat it.

Danggui Sini Decoction (当归四逆汤, Chinese angelica decoction for resolving four kinds of adverseness) [is composed of] 3 *liang* of Danggui (当归, Chinese angelica, Radix Angelicae Sinensis), 3 *liang* of Guizhi (桂枝, cinnamon twig, Ramulus Cinnamomi) (remove the bark), 3 *liang* of Shaoyao (芍药, peony, Radix Paeoniae), 2 *liang* of Gancao (甘草, licorice, Radix Glycyrrhizae Praeparata) (broil), 2 *liang* of Tongcao (通草, rice-paper plant pith, Medulla Tetrapanacis) and 25 pieces of Dazao (大枣, jujube, Fructus Ziziphus Jujubae) (break).

These seven ingredients are decocted in 8 *sheng* of water to get 3 *sheng* [after boiling]. The dregs are removed and [the decoction is] taken warm 1 *sheng* [each time] and three times a day.

【英译】

Line 352

If [there is] internal cold in the patient for a long time, Danggui Sini Decoction (当归四逆汤, Chinese angelica decoction for resolving four kinds of adverseness) added with Wuzhuyu Shengjiang Decoction (吴茱萸生姜汤, evodia and ginger decoction) should [be used to treat it].

Wuzhuyu Shengjiang Decoction (吴茱萸生姜汤, evodia and ginger decoction) [is composed of] 2 *liang* of Danggui (当归, Chinese angelica, Radix Angelicae Sinesis), 3 *liang* of Shaoyao (芍药, peony, Radix Paeoniae), 2 *liang* of Gancao (甘草, licorice, Radix Glycyrrhizae Praeparata) (broil), 2 *liang* of Tongcao (通草, rice-paper plant pith, Medulla Tetrapanacis), 3 *liang* of Guizhi (桂枝, cinnamon twig, Radix Glycyrrhizae Praeparata) (remove the bark), 3 *liang* of Xixin (细辛, asarum, Herba Asari), 0.5 *jin* of Shengjiang (生姜, fresh ginger, Rhizoma Zingiberis Recens) (cut), 2 *sheng* of Wuzhuyu (吴茱萸, evodia, Fructus Euodiae) and 25 pieces of Dazao (大枣, jujube, Fructus Ziziphus Jujubae) (break).

These nine ingredients are decocted in 6 *sheng* of water mixed with 6 *sheng* of clear wine to get 5 *sheng* [after] boiling. The dregs are removed and [the decoction is] divided into five [doses] and taken warm. Another edition [says that there is] 4 *sheng* of water and wine respectively.

【原文】

(三五三)

大汗出,热不去,内拘急,四肢疼,又下利厥逆而恶寒者,四逆汤主之。

【今译】

患者大汗淋漓,但热仍不退,腹中拘急,四肢疼痛,又有腹泻,四肢厥冷,恶寒,宜用四逆汤主治。

【原文】

(三五四)

大汗,若大下利而厥冷者,四逆汤主之。

【今译】

大汗出后,如果有严重的腹泻,且手足厥冷的,用四逆汤主治。

【原文】

(三五五)

病人手足厥冷,脉乍紧者,邪结在胸中,心下满而烦,饥不能食者,病在胸中,当须吐之,宜瓜蒂散。

【今译】

如果病人手足厥冷,脉象忽然紧者,为实邪结在胸中所致,心下胀满烦躁,虽然饥饿却不能进食,说明病在胸中,应当用涌吐法治疗,宜用瓜蒂散主治。

Differentiation of pulse and syndrome/pattern [related to] jueyin disease and treatment

【英译】

Line 353

[In this disease, there are symptoms and signs of] incessant presence of heat after profuse sweating, heat, internal spasm, pain of the four limbs, diarrhea, reversal [cold of limbs] and adversion to cold. Sini Decoction (四逆汤, decoction for resolving four kinds of adverseness) [can be used] to treat it.

【英译】

Line 354

[After] profuse sweating, if there is severe diarrhea with reversal cold [of limbs], [it can be] treated by Sini Decoction (四逆汤, decoction for resolving four kinds of adverseness).

【英译】

Line 355

[If there is] reversal cold of hands and feet with suddenly tight pulse in the patient, [it is caused by] pagthogenic factors binding in the chest, [accompanied by] fullness and vexation below the heart, hunger without ability to eat, [indicating that] the disease is in the chest and should [be treated by] vomiting [therapy]. The appropriate [formula] is Guadi Powder (瓜蒂散, melon stalk powder).

【原文】

(三五六)

伤寒,厥而心下悸,宜先治水,当服茯苓甘草汤,却治其厥。不尔,水渍入胃,必作利也。

【今译】

伤寒病,患者四肢厥冷,心下悸动,宜先治其水饮,当服茯苓甘草汤,然后再治其厥。不这样治疗,水饮就会浸渍肠胃,必然导致腹泻。

【原文】

(三五七)

伤寒六七日,大下后,寸脉沉而迟,手足厥逆,下部脉不至,喉咽不利,唾脓血,泄利不止者,为难治,麻黄升麻汤主之。

麻黄升麻汤方

麻黄二两半(去节)、升麻一两一分、当归一两一分、知母十八铢、黄芩十八铢、葳蕤十八铢(一作菖蒲)、芍药六铢、天门冬六铢(去心)、桂枝六铢(去皮)、茯苓六铢、甘草六铢(炙)、石膏六铢(碎,绵裹)、白术六铢、干姜六铢。

右十四味,以水一斗,先煮麻黄一两沸,去上沫,内诸药,煮取三升,去滓,分温三服,相去如炊三斗米顷,令尽,汗出愈。

【今译】

伤寒病发作六七天,用峻下法治疗后,出现寸脉沉而迟、手足厥冷、尺脉不现、咽喉疼痛、吞咽困难、唾吐脓血、腹泻不止等症状,为难治之症,宜用麻黄升麻汤主治。

Differentiation of pulse and syndrome/pattern [related to] jueyin disease and treatment

【英译】

Line 356

[In] cold damage [disease], [there is] reversal [cold of limbs] with palpitation. [It is] appropriate to treat water [retention] first with [the formula of] Fuling Gancao Decoction (茯苓甘草汤, poria and licorice decoction). Then reversal [cold of limbs] should be treated. [If] not [treated in such a way], water will soak into the stomach and inevitably cause diarrhea.

【英译】

Line 357

Six or seven days [after occurrence of] cold damage [disease], [it is treated by] drastic purgation, [the following symptoms and signs include] sunken and slow pulse in the cun [region], reversal [cold] of hands and feet, insensible pulse in the lower region (chi pulse), sore-throat, difficulty in swallowing, vomiting of pus and blood and incessant diarrhea, very difficult to treat. Mahuang Shengma Decoction (麻黄升麻汤, ephedra and cimicifuga decoction) [can be used] to treat it.

Mahuang Shengma Decoction (麻黄升麻汤, ephedra and cimicifuga decoction) [is composed of] 2.5 *liang* of Mahuang (麻黄, ephedra, Herba Ephedrae) (remove the nodes), 1 *liang* and 1 *fen* of Shengma (升麻, cimicifuga, Rhizoma Cimicifugae), 1 *liang* and 1 *fen* of Danggui (当归, Chinese angelica, Radix Angelicae Sinensis), 18 *zhu* of Zhimu (知母, rhizome of common anemarrhena, Rhizoma Anemarrhenae), 18 *zhu* of Huangqin (黄芩, scutellaria, Radix Scutellariae), 18 *zhu* of Weirui (葳蕤, solomon's seed, Rhizoma Polygonati Odorati), 6 *zhu* of Shaoyao (芍药, peony, Radix Paeoniae), 6 *zhu* of Tianmendong (天门冬, asparagus, Radix Asparagus), 6 *zhu* of Guizhi (桂枝, cinnamon twig, Ramulus Cinnamomi) (remove the bark), 6 *zhu* of Gancao (甘草, licorice, Radix Glycyrrhizae Praeparata) (broil), 6 *zhu* of Shigao (石膏, gypsum, Gypsum Fibrosum) (crush and wrap in the gauze), 6 *zhu* of Baizhu (白术, rhizome of largeheaded atractylodes, Rhizoma Atractylodes Macrocephala) and 6 *zhu* of Ganjiang (干姜, dried ginger, Rhizoma Zingiberis).

These fourteen ingredients are decocted in 1 *dou* of water. Mahuang (麻黄, ephedra, Herba Ephedrae) is boiled first for once or twice. The foam is removed and other ingredients are put into it to boil and get 3 *sheng*. The dregs are removed and [the decoction is] divided into three [doses] and taken warm. [The decoction is finished] in the same way as cooking 3 *dou* of rice. [When the decoction is] completely taken and sweating issues, [the disease will] heal.

【原文】

(三五八)

伤寒四五日,腹中痛,若转气下趣少腹者,此欲自利也。

【今译】

伤寒病发作四五天后,患者腹中疼痛,如果腹内气转动下行到小腹,即将引起腹泻。

【原文】

(三五九)

伤寒本自寒下,医复吐下之,寒格,更逆吐下,若食入口即吐,干姜黄芩黄连人参汤主之。

干姜黄芩黄连人参汤方

干姜、黄芩、黄连、人参各三两。

右四味,以水六升,煮取两升,去滓,分温再服。

【今译】

伤寒病本来因虚寒而导致腹泻,医生则误用吐法和下法治疗,以致虚寒更甚,吐泻严重。如果饮食入口即吐,可用干姜黄芩黄连人参汤主治。

Differentiation of pulse and syndrome/pattern [related to] jueyin disease and treatment

【英译】

Line 358

Four or five days [after occurrence of] cold damage [disease], [there is] abdominal pain. If qi [in the abdomen] descends towards the lower abdomen, it will cause diarrhea.

【英译】

Line 359

[In] cold damage [disease], diarrhea [is caused by] cold. [But] doctor has [treated it with] vomiting and purgation [therapies], [making] cold more serious. Further adverse [treatment] will aggravate vomiting and diarrhea. Ganjiang Huangqin Huanglian Renshen Decoction (干姜黄芩黄连人参汤, dried ginger, scutellaria, coptis and ginseng decoction) [can be used] to treat it.

Ganjiang Huangqin Huanglian Renshen Decoction (干姜黄芩黄连人参汤, dried ginger, scutellaria, coptis and ginseng decoction) [is composed of] 3 *liang* of Ganjiang (干姜, dried ginger, Rhizoma Zingiberis), 3 *liang* of Huangqin (黄芩, scutellaria, Radix Scutellariae), 3 *liang* of Huanglian (黄连, coptis, Rhizoma Coptidis) and 3 *liang* of Renshen (人参, ginseng, Radix Ginseng).

These four ingredients are decocted in 6 *sheng* of water to get 2 *sheng* [after] boiling. The dregs are removed and [the decoction is] divided [into two doses] and taken warm.

【原文】

(三六〇)

下利,有微热而渴,脉弱者,今自愈。

【今译】

患者腹泻,轻微发热,口渴,脉象弱,即将痊愈。

【原文】

(三六一)

下利脉数,有微热汗出,今自愈。设复紧,为未解。

【今译】

腹泻,脉数,轻度发热汗出,病即将痊愈。假如脉象又紧,说明病仍未解。

【原文】

(三六二)

下利,手足厥冷,无脉者,灸之。不温,若脉不还,反微喘者,死。少阴负跌阳者,为顺也。

【今译】

腹泻,手足厥冷,脉搏不跳,需以灸法回阳复脉。如果灸后手足仍不温暖,脉搏仍不跳动,反有微喘症状的,属于死候。如果足部的太溪脉小于跌阳脉,属顺症。

Differentiation of pulse and syndrome/pattern [related to] jueyin disease and treatment

【英译】

Line 360

[In this disease, there are symptoms and signs of] diarrhea, slight fever, thirst and weak pulse, [indicating that the disease is] about to heal spontaneously [because pathogenic factors have declined and yang qi is restored].

【英译】

Line 361

[The symptoms and signs of] diarrhea, rapid pulse, mild fever and sweating [indicate that] the disease is about to heal. If [the pulse is] again tight, [the disease is] not yet resolved.

【英译】

Line 362

[The disease with the symptoms and signs of] diarrhea, reversal cold of hands and feet and absence of pulse, moxibustion [can be used to treat] it [in order to restore yang and pulse]. [After application of moxibustion, if hands and feet are still] not warm, and if the pulse is still absent, but [there is] mild panting, [it is] fatal. [If] shaoyin (kidney meridian, the pulsation of which is at Taixi, the third acupoint located on this meridian) is lesser than Fuyang (stomach meridian, the pulsation of which is at Chongyang, the forty-second acupoint located on this meridian), [it is] favourable.

【原文】

(三六三)

下利,寸脉反浮数,尺中自涩者,必清脓血。

【今译】

腹泻,寸脉反而浮数,尺脉则自涩,大便必下脓血。

【原文】

(三六四)

下利清谷,不可攻表,汗出必胀满。

【今译】

腹泻,完谷不化,不可通过发汗以攻解表。如果使用发汗法,必然引起腹部胀满。

【原文】

(三六五)

下利,脉沉弦者,下重也。脉大者,为未止;脉微弱数者,为欲自止,虽发热,不死。

【今译】

腹泻,脉沉弦的,有后重之感。如果脉象大,说明腹泻还在继续。如果脉象微弱而数,说明腹泻将要自愈。虽然患者发热,但并不危险。

Differentiation of pulse and syndrome/pattern [related to] jueyin disease and treatment

【英译】

Line 363

[In this disease, there is] diarrhea, the cun pulse is floating and rapid, the chi pulse is spontaneously rough. [Consequently] there will be stool with pus and blood.

【英译】

Line 364

[In this disease,] diarrhea with undigested food cannot [be resolved by] attacking the external [by means of diaphoresis], [because] sweating will cause [abdominal] distension and fullness.

【英译】

Line 365

[If there is] diarrhea and sunken and taut pulse, [it indicates] tenesmus. Large pulse indicates [that diarrhea] does not cease. Faint, weak and rapid pulse indicates [that it will] spontaneously cease. Although there is fever, [the patient] will not die.

【原文】

(三六六)

下利,脉沉而迟,其人面少赤,身有微热,下利清谷者,必郁冒汗出而解,病人必微厥。所以然者,其面戴阳,下虚故也。

【今译】

腹泻,脉象沉而迟,患者面部微红,体表有微热,下利清谷,汗出而病解的现象一定会出现,患者四肢轻微厥冷。之所以如此,是因为面戴阳,下部虚所致。

【原文】

(三六七)

下利,脉数而渴者,今自愈。设不差,必清脓血,以有热故也。

【今译】

腹泻,脉数而口渴,说明疾病即将自愈。假如不愈,必然发生大便脓血,原因是里有热邪。

Differentiation of pulse and syndrome / pattern [related to] jueyin disease and treatment

【英译】

Line 366

[The disease is characterized by] diarrhea, sunken and slow pulse, slightly red face, mild fever and diarrhea with undigested food. [The disease is eventually] resolved through sweating and there is mild reversal [cold in] the patient. The reason [is that there is] yang in the face (red color, indicating decline of yang qi) and deficiency of the lower [part of the body].

【英译】

Line 367

[In this disease,] diarrhea with rapid pulse and thirst [indicates that the disease is] about to heal spontaneously. If [the disease is] not cured, there will be pus and blood in the stool due to heat.

【原文】

(三六八)

下利后脉绝,手足厥冷,晬时脉还,手足温者生,脉不还者死。

【今译】

腹泻后摸不到脉搏,手足厥冷,一昼夜后脉搏恢复,手足变温的,可以治愈。如果脉搏仍不恢复,则无生还希望。

【原文】

(三六九)

伤寒,下利,日十余行,脉反实者,死。

【今译】

伤寒,腹泻,一日十多次,脉搏反而有力的,为死候。

【原文】

(三七〇)

下利清谷,里寒外热,汗出而厥者,通脉四逆汤主之。

【今译】

腹泻,完谷不化,里寒外热、汗出而四肢厥冷的,用通脉四逆汤主治。

Differentiation of pulse and syndrome/pattern [related to] jueyin disease and treatment

【英译】

Line 368

After diarrhea, the pulse is insensible, hands and feet are reversally cold. [After] one day and one night, the pulse returns, hands and feet are warm, [indicating that the disease is] curable. [If] the pulse does not return, [it is] fatal.

【英译】

Line 369

[In] cold damage [disease], [there is] diarrhea for more than ten times a day, but the pulse is strong, [indicating that it is] fatal.

【英译】

Line 370

[Disease, characterized by] diarrhea with undigested food, internal cold and external heat, sweating and reversal [cold of limbs], [can be] treated by Tongmai Sini Decoction (通脉四逆汤, decoction for freeing meridians and resolving four kinds of adverseness).

【原文】

(三七一)

热利下重者,白头翁汤主之。

白头翁汤方

白头翁二两、黄柏三两、黄连三两、秦皮三两。

右四味,以水七升,煮取两升,去滓,温服一升。不愈,更服一升。

【今译】

热症下利,里急后重的,用白头翁汤主治。

【原文】

(三七二)

下利腹胀满,身体疼痛者,先温其里,乃攻其表。温里宜四逆汤,攻表宜桂枝汤。

【今译】

腹泻,腹部胀满,身体疼痛的,应先温其里,然后再解其表。温里宜用四逆汤,解表宜用桂枝汤。

Differentiation of pulse and syndrome／pattern ［related to］ jueyin disease and treatment

【英译】

Line 371

［The disease characterized by］ heat，diarrhea and tenesmus ［can be］ treated by Baitouweng Decoction（白头翁汤，pulsatilla decoction）.

Baitouweng Decoction（白头翁汤，pulsatilla decoction）［is composed of］ 2 *liang* of Baitouweng（白头翁，pulsatilla，Radix Pulsatillae），3 *liang* of Huangbo（黄柏，phellodendron，Cortex Phellodendri Chinensis），3 *liang* of Huanglian（黄连，coptis，Rhizoma Coptidis）and 3 *liang* of Qinpi（秦皮，the bark of ash，Cortex Fraxini）.

These four ingredients are decocted in 7 *sheng* of water and get 2 *sheng* ［after］ boiling. The dregs are removed and ［the decoction is］ taken warm 1 *sheng* ［each time］. ［If the disease is］ not cured，take another *sheng* ［of decoction］.

【英译】

Line 372

［When there are symptoms and signs of］ diarrhea，abdominal distension and fullness and generalized pain，［it should be treated by］ warming the internal first and then resolving the external. To warm the internal，Sini Decoction（四逆汤，decoction for resolving four kinds of adverseness）should be used. To resolve the external，Guizhi Decoction（桂枝汤，cinnamon twig decoction）should be used.

【原文】

(三七三)

下利,欲饮水者,以有热故也。白头翁汤主之。

【今译】

腹泻,口渴欲饮水,是因为其里有热,用白头翁汤主治。

【原文】

(三七四)

下利谵语者,有燥屎也。宜小承气汤。

【今译】

腹泻兼谵语的,是肠中燥屎所致,宜用小承气汤治疗。

【原文】

(三七五)

下利后,更烦,按之心下濡者,为虚烦也,宜栀子豉汤。

【今译】

腹泻以后,患者更加心烦,心下部按之柔软,此为虚烦之症,宜用栀子豉汤主治。

Differentiation of pulse and syndrome/pattern [related to] jueyin disease and treatment

【英译】

Line 373

Diarrhea with thirst and desire to drink water is [caused by] heat in the internal. Baitouweng Decoction (白头翁汤, pulsatilla decoction) [can be used] to treat it.

【英译】

Line 374

Diarrhea with delirium [is caused by] dry stool [in the intestines]. Xiao Chengqi Decoction (小承气汤, minor decoction for harmonizing qi) is the appropriate [formula for treating it].

【英译】

Line 375

After diarrhea, [there is] more vexation and [the region] below the heart is pressed soft. This is deficiency vexation [syndrome/pattern]. Zhizi Chi Decoction (栀子豉汤, gardenia and fermented soybean decoction) is the appropriate [formula for treating it].

【原文】

(三七六)

呕家有痈脓者,不可治呕,脓尽自愈。

【今译】

呕吐的病人,内有痈脓,不应见呕止呕,而应解毒排脓,脓尽则病自愈。

【原文】

(三七七)

呕而脉弱,小便复利,身有微热,见厥者难治,四逆汤主之。

【今译】

患者呕吐而脉弱,小便反而清利,身上轻度发热,如手足厥冷,则难治。用四逆汤治疗。

【原文】

(三七八)

干呕,吐涎沫,头痛者,吴茱萸汤主之。

【今译】

患者干呕,吐涎沫,头痛,用吴茱萸汤主治。

Differentiation of pulse and syndrome / pattern [related to] jueyin disease and treatment

【英译】

Line 376

[In] the patient with retching, there is abscess and suppuration. [Treatment of such a disease should] not focus on retching. [Only when] suppuration is eliminated can [the disease] heal spontaneously.

【英译】

Line 377

[When there is] retching, the pulse is weak, urination is smooth, there is mild fever. If [there is] reversal [cold of limbs], [it is] difficult to treat. Sini Decoction (四逆汤, decoction for resolving four kinds of adverseness) is the appropriate [formula for] treating it.

【英译】

Line 378

[When there are symptoms and signs of] dry retching, vomiting of drool with foam and headache, Wuzhuyu Decoction (吴茱萸汤, evodia decoction) [can be used] to treat it.

【原文】

(三七九)

呕而发热者,小柴胡汤主之。

【今译】

呕吐而见发热的,用小柴胡汤主治。

【原文】

(三八〇)

伤寒,大吐、大下之,极虚,复极汗者,其人外气怫郁,复与之水,以发其汗,因得哕。所以然者,胃中寒冷故也。

【今译】

伤寒病,若用大吐、大下之法,将导致患者身体极其虚弱。如果再急用汗法,患者外气将郁结。然后用水疗法发汗,引起呃逆。之所以如此,是因为胃中寒冷的缘故。

【原文】

(三八一)

伤寒,哕而腹满,视其前后,知何部不利,利之即愈。

【今译】

伤寒病,患者哕逆,腹部胀满。察看其大小便,就能知道何处不通利,只要通利了,病就可以痊愈了。

Differentiation of pulse and syndrome/pattern [related to] jueyin disease and treatment

【英译】

Line 379

[When there is] retching with fever，Xiao Chaihu Decoction
(小柴胡汤，minor bupleurum decoction) [can be used] to treat it.

【英译】

Line 380

[In] cold damage [disease], [application of] great vomiting
and great purgation [therapies will cause] extreme deficiency. [If]
urgent diaphoresis [is used], external qi [will be] stagnated. The
reason is that [there is] cold in the stomach.

【英译】

Line 381

[In] cold damage [disease, there are symptoms and signs of]
hiccup，abdominal distension and fullness. Observation of the front
(urination) and back (defecation) [will enable one] to know which
is inhibited. [Only when it is] disinhibited can [the disease be]
cured.

辨霍乱病脉证并治

(三八二)

问曰：病有霍乱者何？答曰：呕吐而利，此名霍乱。

【今译】

问：什么叫霍乱？

答：呕吐与腹泻并作，称为霍乱。

【原文】

(三八三)

问曰：病发热头痛，身疼恶寒，吐利者，此属何病？答曰：此名霍乱。霍乱自吐下，又利止，复更发热也。

【今译】

问：病有发热头痛，身疼恶寒，呕吐泄泻的，属于什么病？

答：此病称作霍乱。霍乱既自行吐泻，又有腹泻停止，再度发热。

Differentiation of pulse and syndrome/ pattern [related to] cholera and treatment

【英译】

Line 382

Question: What is huoluan (sudden turmoil)?

Answer: [The disease marked by] vomiting and diarrhea is known as huoluan (sudden turmoil).

【英译】

Line 383

Question: What is the disease [characterized by] fever, headache, generalized pain, aversion to cold, vomiting and diarrhea?

Answer: This [disease] is called huoluan (sudden turmoil) [marked by] spontaneous vomiting and diarrhea. [When] diarrhea ceases, fever is more acute.

伤寒论英译

【原文】

(三八四)

伤寒,其脉微涩者,本是霍乱,今是伤寒,却四五日,至阴经上,转入阴必利;本呕,下利者,不可治也。欲似大便,而反失气,仍不利者,此属阳明也。便必鞭,十三日愈。所以然者,经尽故也。下利后,当便鞭,鞭则能食者愈。今反不能食,到后经中,颇能食,复过一经能食,过之一日当愈;不愈者,不属阳明也。

【今译】

伤寒病,其脉象微涩的,本来是霍乱,如今则是伤寒。到了第四五日的时候,就传入阴经,传入阴必然引起腹泻。原本有呕吐和腹泻症状的,无法治疗。患者想大便,反而排气,并且仍然腹泻的,属于阳明证。这时的大便必硬,十三日后可以治愈。之所以如此,是因为病邪已在经中传遍。腹泻后,大便应当硬。大便硬,但患者能进食的,就可以治愈。如今患者反而不能食,当传入到另外一经中,却很能进食。当传入另一经反而能进食,再过一天就应该能治愈了。如果还治不愈的,就不属于阳明证了。

Differentiation of pulse and syndrome/ pattern [related to] sudden turmoil

【英译】

Line 384

Cold damage [disease] with faint and rough pulse originally is huoluan (sudden turmoil). Now it is cold damage [disease]. [But] on the fourth or fifth day, [it will transmit] to the yin meridian. [When it has] transmitted to the yin [meridian], there must be diarrhea. Originally [there is] retching, [but if there is] diarrhea, [it is] difficult to treat. [When the patient] feels to defecate, but [it is] just flatus and [there is] still diarrhea, it belongs to yangming [syndrome/pattern]. [In such a case,] the stool must be hard and [it will be] cured in thirteen days. The reason is that [the pathogenic factors have] already transmitted to the whole meridian. After diarrhea, the stool should be hard. [When the stool is] hard, [the patient is] able to eat and it could be cured. [But] now [the patient is] unable to eat. [When the pathogenic factors have] transmitted to another meridian, [the patient is] quite able to eat. [When the pathogenic factors have] transmitted to the third meridian and [the patient is] able to eat, [the disease will be] cured the next day. [If the disease is] not cured, [it does] not belong to yangming [syndrome/pattern].

【原文】

(三八五)

恶寒,脉微而复利,利止,亡血也。四逆加人参汤主之。

四逆加人参汤方

甘草二两(炙)、附子一枚(生,去皮,破八片)、干姜一两半、人参一两。

右四味,以水三升,煮取一升二合,去滓,分温再服。

【今译】

恶寒,脉象虚微而又腹泻,腹泻停止,则血液耗散,宜用四逆加人参汤治疗。

【原文】

(三八六)

霍乱,头痛,发热,身疼痛,热多欲饮水者,五苓散主之。寒多不用水者,理中丸主之。

理中丸方

人参、干姜、甘草(炙)、白术各三两。

右四味,捣筛,蜜和为丸,如鸡子黄许大。以沸汤数合,和一丸,研碎,温服之,日三四,夜两服。腹中未热,益至三四丸,然不及汤。汤

Differentiation of pulse and syndrome /
pattern [related to] sudden turmoil

【英译】

Line 385

[The disease is characterized by] aversion to cold, thin pulse and diarrhea. [If] diarrhea ceases, there will be blood collapse. The appropriate [formula used] to treat [it is] Sini Decoction (四逆汤, decoction for resolving four kinds of adverseness) added with Renshen (人参, ginseng, Radix Ginseng).

Sini Decoction (四逆汤, decoction for resolving four kinds of adverseness) added with Renshen (人参, ginseng, Radix Ginseng) [is composed of] 2 *liang* of Gancao (甘草, licorice, Radix Glycyrrhea Praeparata) (broil), 1 piece of Fuzi (附子, aconite, Radix Aconiti Lateralis Preparata) (raw, remove the bark and break into eight small pieces), 1. 5 *liang* of Ganjiang (干姜, dried ginger, Rhizoma Zingiberis) and 1 *liang* of Renshen (人参, ginseng, Radix Ginseng).

These four ingredients are decocted in 3 *sheng* of water to get 1. 2 *sheng* [after] boiling. The dregs are removed and [the decoction is] divided [into two doses] and taken warm.

【英译】

Line 386

Huoluan (sudden turmoil) [is characterized by] headache, fever, generalized pain, exuberant heat and desire to drink water. Wuling Powder (五苓散, powder made of five medicinal herbs) [can be used] to treat it. [If there is] exuberant cold and [the patient] does not want to drink water, Lizhong Pill (理中丸, pill for regulating the middle) [can be used] to treat it.

Lizhong Pill (理中丸, pill for regulating the middle) [is composed of] 3 *liang* of Renshen (人参, ginseng, Ginseng), 3 *liang* of Ganjiang (干姜, dried ginger, Rhizoma Zingiberis), 3 *liang* of Baizhu (白术, rhizome of largehead atractylodes, Rhizoma Atractylodis Ovatae) and 3 liang of Gancao (甘草, licorice, Radix Glycyrrhea Praeparata).

These four ingredients are pounded, sieved and mixed with honey [to make into] pills as big as [a chicken's] egg yolk. [Usually] one pill is pounded and boiled in several *ge* of water, [which is] taken warm, three or four times in the daytime and twice at night. [If there is] no heat in the abdomen, three or four more pills [should be taken]. [But such a proceeding way is] not as

法,以四物依两数切,用水八升,煮取三升,去滓,温服一升,日三服。若脐上筑者,肾气动也,去术,加桂四两;吐多者,去术,加生姜三两;下多者,还用术;悸者,加茯苓二两;渴欲得水者,加术,足前成四两半;腹中痛者,加人参,足前成四两半;寒者,加干姜,足前成四两半;腹满者,去术,加附子一枚。服汤后,如食顷,饮热粥一升许,微自温,勿发揭衣被。

【今译】

霍乱病,吐泻,头痛发热,身疼痛,表热较甚而患者想喝水的,宜用五苓散主治。如果寒盛而患者不想喝水,宜用理中丸主治。

【原文】

(三八七)

吐利止而身痛不休者,当消息和解其外,宜桂枝汤小和之。

【今译】

患者呕吐,腹泻停止,身体疼痛不解的,应当斟酌使用解表法,宜用桂枝汤微加和解。

effective as that of the decoction. [As to] the decoction, four ingredients of the amounts mentioned above are cut, decocted in 8 *sheng* of water to get 3 *sheng* [after] boiling. The dregs are removed and [the decoction is] taken warm 1 *sheng* [each time] and three times a day. If [there is] vibration above the navel, kidney qi is stirred. [In this case,] Baizhu (白术, rhizome of largehead atractylodes, Rhizoma Atractylodis Ovatae) [should be] removed and 4 *liang* of Guizhi (桂枝, cinnamon twig, *Ramulus Cinnamomi*) [should be] added. [If there is] excessive vomiting, Baizhu (白术, rhizome of largehead atractylodes, Rhizoma Atractylodis Ovatae) [should be] removed and 3 *liang* of Shengjiang (生姜, fresh ginger, Rhizoma Zingiberis Recens) [should be] added. [If there is] excessive diarrhea, Baizhu (白术, rhizome of largehead atractylodes, Rhizoma Atractylodis Ovatae) still [should be] used. [If there is] palpitation, 2 *liang* of Fuling (茯苓, poria, Poria) [should be] added. [If the patient feels] thirsty and wants to drink water, Baizhu (白术, rhizome of largehead atractylodes, Rhizoma Atractylodis Ovatae) [should be] added, the previous amount [mentioned above should be increased] to 4.5 *liang*. [If there is] abdominal pain, Renshen (人参, ginseng, Ginseng) [should be] added, the previous amount [mentioned above should be increased] to 4.5 *liang*. [If] there is cold, Ganjiang (干姜, dried ginger, Rhizoma Zingiberis) [should be] added, the previous amount [mentioned above should be increased] to 4.5 *liang*. [If there is] abdominal fullness, Baizhu (白术, rhizome of largehead atractylodes, Rhizoma Atractylodis Ovatae) [should be] removed and 1 piece of Fuzi (附子, aconite, Radix Aconiti) [should be] added. After taking the decoction and if [there is a need] to take food, wait for a while and take 1 *sheng* of hot porridge to slightly warm the body, but do not remove the clothes and quilt [when feeling warm].

【英译】

Line 387

[The disease is characterized by] vomiting, diarrhea that does not cease and generalized pain that is not resolved, cares should be taken to harmonize and resolve the external. The appropriate [formula used] to treat it [is] Guizhi Decoction (桂枝汤, cinnamon twig decoction).

【原文】

(三八八)

吐利,汗出,发热,恶寒,四肢拘急,手足厥冷者,四逆汤主之。

【今译】

患者呕吐又腹泻,出汗则发热,同时有恶寒、四肢拘急、手足厥冷等症状,宜用四逆汤主治。

【原文】

(三八九)

既吐且利,小便复利而大汗出,下利清谷,内寒外热,脉微欲绝者,四逆汤主之。

【今译】

患者既呕吐,又腹泻,小便通畅,大汗淋漓,下利清谷,体内有寒,体表发热,脉微弱至极,宜用四逆汤主治。

Differentiation of pulse and syndrome/ pattern [related to] sudden turmoil

【英译】

Line 388

[The disease, characterized by] vomiting, diarrhea, fever, aversion to cold, spasm of limbs and reversal cold of hands and feet, should be treated by Sini Decoction (四逆汤, decoction for resolving four kinds of adverseness).

【英译】

Line 389

[The disease, characterized by] vomiting, diarrhea, normal defecation, profuse sweating, sloppy stool with undigested food, internal cold and external heat, faint pulse about to disappear, should be treated by Sini Decoction (四逆汤, decoction for resolving four kinds of adverseness).

【原文】

(三九〇)

吐已下断,汗出而厥,四肢拘急不解,脉微欲绝者,通脉四逆加猪胆汁汤主之。

通脉四逆加猪胆汤方

甘草二两(炙)、干姜三两(强人可四两)、附子大者一枚(生,去皮,破八片)、猪胆汁半合。

右四味,以水三升,煮取一升二合,去滓,内猪胆汁,分温再服,其脉即来。无猪胆,以羊胆代之。

【今译】

吐下虽然停止,但汗出后则出现厥冷,四肢拘急不解,脉象虚微欲绝,宜用通脉四逆加猪汁汤主治。

【原文】

(三九一)

吐利,发汗,脉平,小烦者,以新虚不胜谷气故也。

【今译】

患者呕吐,腹泻,发汗后脉搏平和,但却略感觉烦躁,这是因为发病后出现新的虚证,从而使脾胃之气虚弱所致。

Differentiation of pulse and syndrome/ pattern [related to] sudden turmoil

【英译】

Line 390

Although vomiting is ceased, but reversal [cold appears after] sweating, the spasm of the limbs is not resolved, and the pulse is faint and about to disappear. [It should be] treated by Tongmai Sini Decoction (通脉四逆汤, decoction for freeing vessels and resolving four kinds of adverseness) added with Zhudanzhi (猪胆汁, pig's bile, Suis Bilis).

Tongmai Sini Decoction (通脉四逆汤, decoction for freeing vessels and resolving four kinds of adverseness) added with Zhudanzhi (猪胆汁, pig's bile, Suis Bilis) [is composed of] 2 *liang* of Gancao (甘草, licorice, Radix Glycyrrhizae Praeparata) (broil), 3 *liang* (4 *liang* for those who are strong) of Ganjiang (干姜, dried ginger, Rhizoma Zingiberis),1 piece of Fuzi (附子, aconite, Radix Aconiti Laterlis Preparata) (raw, remove the bark and break into eight small pieces), and 0.5 *ge* of Zhudanzhi (猪胆汁, pig's bile, Suis Bilis).

These four ingredients are decocted in 3 *sheng* of water to get 1 *sheng* and 2 *ge* [after] boiling. The dregs are removed, Zhudanzhi (猪胆汁, pig's bile, Suis Bilis) is put into [it]. [The decoction is] divided [into two doses] and taken warm. [After taking the decoction,] the pulse will begin to beat. [If there is] no pig's bile, sheep's bile can replace it.

【英译】

Line 391

[The disease is characterized by] vomiting and diarrhea. [After] sweating, the pulse [becomes] calm, [but the patient feels] somewhat vexing. [This is] due to new deficiency [syndrome/pattern after occurrence of the disease, making] stomach and spleen qi [weak].

辨阴阳易差后劳复病脉证并治

【原文】

(三九二)

伤寒阴阳易之为病,其人身体重,少气,少腹里急,或引阴中拘挛,热上冲胸,头重不欲举,眼中生花,膝胫拘急者,烧裈散主之。

烧裈散方

妇人中裈近隐处,取烧作灰。

右一味,水服方寸匕,日三服,小便即利,阴头微肿,此为愈矣。妇人病,取男子裈烧服。

【今译】

伤寒病后,阴阳变易而发病,其临床表现为身体沉重,气少不足以息,小腹挛急,或牵引阴部挛急,热气上冲至胸,头重不能抬起,眼睛发花,膝部与小腿肚拘急,宜用烧裈散治疗。

Differentiation of yin and yang, examination of pulse and treatment of syndrome/pattern

【英译】

Line 392

[In] cold damage [disease], exchange of yin and yang [will cause disease with the symptoms and signs of] heaviness of the body, shortness of breath, spasm in the lower abdomen, or spasm involving the genitals, heat running into the chest, heaviness of the head with no desire to raise, blurred vision and spasm of the knees and lower leg. [It can be] treated by Shaokun Powder (烧裈散, powder for burning pants).

Shaokun Powder (烧裈散, powder for burning pants) is managed in the following way.

Take a part of a woman's pants close to the crotch and burn it into ashes. This ingredient is taken with a *fangcunbi* (about 1 gram) of water, three times a day. [When] urination is normal and glans penis is slightly swollen [after taking the ingredient], [it indicates that] the disease is about to heal. [When] a woman is ill, [she can] take [the powder produced by] burning a man's pants.

【原文】

(三九三)

大病差后,劳复者,枳实栀子豉汤主之。

枳实栀子豉汤方

枳实三枚(炙)、栀子十四个(擘)、香豉一升(绵裹)。

右三味,以清浆水七升,空煮取四升,内枳实、栀子,煮取二升,下豉,更煮五六沸,去滓,温分再服,覆令微似汗。若有宿食者,内大黄如博棋子大五六枚,服之愈。

【今译】

伤寒大病初愈,患者因劳累过度而复发,宜用枳实栀子豉汤主治。

【原文】

(三九四)

伤寒差以后,更发热,小柴胡汤主之。脉浮者,以汗解之;脉沉实者,以下解之。

【今译】

伤寒病痊愈之后,又再次发热,宜用小柴胡汤主治。如果脉浮的,可用发汗法解表祛邪。如果脉沉而有力的,可用攻下法治疗。

Differentiation of yin and yang, examination of pulse and treatment of syndrome / pattern

【英译】

Line 393

After recovery of severe disease [in cold damage disease], [if the patient] works hard [and the disease has] relapsed, Zhishi Zhizichi Decoction (枳实栀子豉汤, processed unripe bitter orange, gardenia and fermented soybean decoction) [can be used] to treat it.

Zhishi Zhizichi Decoction (枳实栀子豉汤, processed unripe bitter orange, gardenia and fermented soybean decoction) [is composed of] 3 pieces of Zhishi (枳实, processed unripe bitter orange, Fructus Aurantii Immaturus) (broil), 14 pieces of Zhizi (栀子, gardenia, Fructus Gardeniae) (break) and 1 *sheng* of Xiangchi (香豉, fermented soybean, Semen Sojae Praeparatum) wrapped in the gauze.

These three ingredients are decocted in 7 *sheng* of clear starch water to get 4 *sheng* [after] boiling without [any other ingredients]. [Then] Zhishi (枳实, processed unripe bitter orange, Fructus Aurantii Immaturus) and Zhizi (栀子, gardenia, Fructus Gardeniae) are put [into it] to boil and get 2 *sheng*. Finally Xiangchi (香豉, fermented soybean, Semen Sojae Praeparatum) is boiled in it for five to six times. The dregs are removed and [the decoction is] divided [into two doses] and taken warm. [After taking the decoction, the patient should] cover [with quilt in order] to induce slight sweating. If there is undigested food [in the stomach], five or six pieces of Dahuang (大黄, rhubarb, Radix et Rhizoma Rhei), about the size of a chess piece, are added. [After] taking [such a decoction], [the disease will be] cured.

【英译】

Line 394

[If] there is fever again after cold damage [disease] is cured, Xiao Chaihu Decoction (小柴胡汤, minor bupleurum decoction) [can be used] to treat it. [If] the pulse is floating, diaphoresis [can be used] to resolve it. [If] the pulse is sunken and strong, purgation [can be used] to resolve it.

【原文】

(三九五)

大病差后,从腰以下有水气者,牡蛎泽泻散主之。

牡蛎泽泻散方

牡蛎(熬)、泽泻、蜀漆(暖水洗去腥)、葶苈子(熬)、商陆根(熬)、海藻(洗去咸)、栝楼根各等分。

右七味,异捣,下筛为散,更于臼中治之,白饮和服方寸匕,日三服,小便利,止后服。

【今译】

伤寒大病痊愈之后,从腰以下有水气的,宜用牡蛎泽泻散主治。

【原文】

(三九六)

大病差后,喜唾,久不了了,胸上有寒,当以丸药温之,宜理中丸。

【今译】

伤寒大病痊愈后,患者总爱泛吐唾沫,始终不能自制,这是因为寒饮停聚胸膈所致,应当用丸药温补,可用理中丸主治。

Differentiation of yin and yang, examination of pulse and treatment of syndrome/pattern

【英译】

Line 395

[If] there is water qi (edema) from the waist downwards after severe disease [in cold damage] is cured, Muli Zexie Powder (牡蛎泽泻散, oyster shell and alisma powder) [can be used] to treat it.

Muli Zexie Powder (牡蛎泽泻散, oyster shell and alisma powder) [is composed of] Muli (牡蛎, oyster shell, Concha Ostreae) (simmer), Zexie (泽泻, alisma, Rhizoma Alismatis), Shuqi (蜀漆, dichroa, Ramulus et Folium Dichroae), Tinglizi (葶苈子, semen tingli, Semen Lepidii seu Descuraniniae) (simmer), Shanglugen (商陆根, phytolacca, Radix Phytolaccae)(simmer), Haizao (海藻, sargassum, Sargassum) and Gualougen (栝楼根, trichosanthes root, Radix Trichosanthes), [which are] of the same amount.

These seven ingredients are pounded separately and sieved into powder. [The powder is put into] a mortar to blend with rice porridge. [The final decoction is] taken 1 *fangcunbi* (about 1 gram) [each time] and three times a day. [When] urination is smooth, stop taking [the decoction].

【英译】

Line 396

After recovery of a severe disease [in cold damage], [the patient is] frequently spitting and [it is] difficult to be resolved [because] there is cold in the chest. [It can be treated] by warming with pills. The appropriate [formula is] Lizhong Pill (理中丸, pill for regulating the middle).

【原文】

(三九七)

伤寒解后,虚羸少气,气逆欲吐,竹叶石膏汤主之。

竹叶石膏汤方

竹叶两把、石膏一斤、半夏半升(洗)、麦门冬一升(去心)、人参三两、甘草二两(炙)、粳米半升。

右七味,以水一斗,煮取六升,去滓,内粳米,煮米熟汤成,去米,温服一升,日三服。

【今译】

伤寒病消解之后,患者身体虚弱消瘦,气息不足,气逆欲吐,宜用竹叶石膏汤主治。

【原文】

(三九八)

病人脉已解,而日暮微烦,以病新差,人强与谷,脾胃气尚弱,不能消谷,故令微烦,损谷则愈。

【今译】

病人病脉已和解,每天傍晚时则有轻微烦闷,这是因为疾病刚缓解,但脾胃还很虚弱,消化能力还差,勉强进食则不能消化,因此而引起轻微烦闷。遇到这种情况,只有减少饮食才能使疾病痊愈。

Differentiation of yin and yang, examination of pulse and treatment of syndrome/pattern

【英译】

Line 397

After resolution of cold damage [disease], [there are still symptoms and signs of] weakness, emaciation, insufficiency of qi, counterflow of qi and nausea. [It can be treated by] Zhuye Shigao Decoction (竹叶石膏汤, bamboo leaf and gypsum decoction).

Zhuye Shigao Decoction (竹叶石膏汤, bamboo leaf and gypsum decoction) [is composed of] 2 bunches of Zhuye (竹叶, bamboo leaf, Herba Lophatheri), 1 *jin* of Shigao (石膏, gypsum, Gypsum Fibrosum), 0.5 *sheng* of Banxia (半夏, Pinellia, Rhizoma Pinelliae) washed, 1 *sheng* of Maimendong (麦门冬, ophiopogon, Rhizoma Ophiopogon) (remove the heart), 3 *liang* of Renshen (人参, ginseng, Radix Ginseng), 2 *liang* of Gancao (甘草, licorice, Radix Glycyrrhizae Praeparata) broiled and 0.5 *sheng* of Jingmi (粳米, polished round-grained rice, Semen Oryzae Nonglutinosae).

These seven ingredients are decocted in 1 *dou* of water to get 6 *sheng* [after] boiling. The dregs are removed and Jingmi (粳米, polished round-grained rice, Semen Oryzae Nonglutinosae) is put into [it] to boil into porridge. [The dregs of] rice are removed and [the decoction is] taken warm 1 *sheng* [each time] and three times a day.

【英译】

Line 398

[The condition of] the patient's pulse is already resolved. But every night, [the patient feels] vexing. [Although] the disease is basically cured, the spleen and stomach are still weak and are difficult to digest food. That is why [the patient feels] vexing [at night]. [Only when] food is decreased [can the disease be] cured.

图书在版编目(CIP)数据

伤寒论英译:英文/(东汉)张仲景著;刘希茹今译;李照国英译.—上海:上海三联书店,2022.8
(国学经典外译丛书.第一辑)
ISBN 978-7-5426-7798-3

Ⅰ.①伤… Ⅱ.①张…②刘…③李… Ⅲ.①《伤寒论》-译文-英文 Ⅳ.①R222.2

中国版本图书馆 CIP 数据核字(2022)第 142547 号

国学经典外译丛书·第一辑

伤寒论英译

著　　者 / (东汉)张仲景
今　　译 / 刘希茹
英　　译 / 李照国
责任编辑 / 杜　鹃
装帧设计 / 徐　徐
监　　制 / 姚　军
责任校对 / 王凌霄

出版发行 / 上海三联书店
　　　　　(200030)中国上海市漕溪北路 331 号 A 座 6 楼
邮　　箱 / sdxsanlian@sina.com
邮购电话 / 021-22895540
印　　刷 / 上海颛辉印刷厂有限公司

版　　次 / 2022 年 8 月第 1 版
印　　次 / 2022 年 8 月第 1 次印刷
开　　本 / 640mm×960mm　1/16
字　　数 / 350 千字
印　　张 / 28.25
书　　号 / ISBN 978-7-5426-7798-3/R·124
定　　价 / 99.00 元

敬启读者,如发现本书有印装质量问题,请与印刷厂联系 021-56152633